Harris A Lewin

MEDICAL
INTELLIGENCE
UNIT

RETROVIRAL LATENCY

Mark A. Laughlin, M.D.
Roger J. Pomerantz, M.D.

Thomas Jefferson University
Division of Infectious Diseases
Philadelphia, Pennsylvania, U.S.A.

R.G. LANDES COMPANY
AUSTIN

MEDICAL INTELLIGENCE UNIT

RETROVIRAL LATENCY

R.G. LANDES COMPANY
Austin

CRC Press is the exclusive worldwide distributor of publications of the Medical Intelligence Unit.
CRC Press, 2000 Corporate Blvd., NW, Boca Raton, FL 33431. Phone: 407/994-0555.

Submitted: September 1994
Published: November 1994

Please address all inquiries to the Publisher:
R.G. Landes Company, 909 Pine Street, Georgetown, TX 78626
or
P.O. Box 4858, Austin, TX 78765
Phone: 512/ 863 7762; FAX: 512/ 863 0081

ISBN 1-57059-034-6
CATALOG # LN9034

To Our Readers

R.G. Landes Company publishes four book series: *Medical Intelligence Unit, Molecular Biology Intelligence Unit, Neuroscience Intelligence Unit,* and *Biotechnology Intelligence Unit.* Our goal is to publish the most recent information in biomedical science for sophisticated researchers and physicians.

To achieve this goal we have accelerated our publishing program to conform to the fast pace in which information grows in biomedical science. The book you have in hand, like all titles in our series, was published *within 90 to 120 days of receipt of the manuscript.*

As you might expect, this causes a few problems for us; sometimes it makes our office more like a big city newspaper than a scholarly publisher. So as you look through this book you may see something that isn't just right. Please let us know. Or if you have an idea for improving our books, we'd like very much to hear from you. If the problem you describe hasn't already been discovered or if your idea is provocative enough to promote a discussion here, we'll give you a free book of your choice. Just list three titles in order of preference and we'll send you one, based on availability—with our thanks. Our address is printed on the copyright page of each of our books.

Carol Harwell
Publications Director
R.G. Landes Company

CONTENTS

CHAPTER 1

OVERVIEW OF RETROVIROLOGY

The recent explosion of research stemming from the worldwide Acquired Immunodeficiency Syndrome (AIDS) epidemic has focused attention on a unique group of viruses, the retroviruses. Their name derives from the ability of these agents to reverse transcribe their genomic RNA into DNA which subsequently serves as the template for further viral production. A second unique feature of these agents which clearly sets them apart from other infectious pathogens is that following reverse transcription, there is integration of the proviral DNA into the infected host cell's genome. This newly acquired cluster of retroviral genes now becomes a permanent part of the infected cell; the fate of the cell isdetermined by both the level of expression from these proviral genes and the influence their presence has upon neighboring cellular genes. The unique life cycle of these pathogens results in a complex host-virus interaction and this complexity is reflected in a wide spectrum of clinical syndromes ranging from totally silent infections to rapidly fatal ones.

While the human immunodeficiency viruses (HIVs) have commanded the majority of public attention, the simian immunodeficiency viruses (SIVs) are providing valuable perspectives into this host-virus interaction. Nearly 50% of African green monkeys are infected with a subspecies of SIV (designated SIVagm) in the wild; and yet no clinical illness has been associated to date.[1-5] Similarly, sooty mangabeys have been shown, both in the wild and in breeding colonies, to be infected with another subspecies of simian immunodeficiency virus designated SIVsm.[6,7] Like the African green monkey infection, the sooty mangabey infection appears to cause no disease in its native host. In one particular breeding colony of sooty mangabeys where the original SIVsm isolate was discovered, as many as 80% of the colony was infected (some for over a decade) without any evidence of disease.[6] Of even greater interest, however, is the striking homology between this SIV of sooty mangabeys and human immunodeficiency virus type 2 (HIV-2) which causes one of the AIDS syndromes in humans.[7-9] In fact, the phylogenetic relatedness between HIV-2 and SIVsm is far greater than between HIV-1 and HIV-2 or between SIVagm and SIVsm.[8-10] The shared geographic distribution of HIV-2 and the natural habitat of sooty mangabeys has fueled the speculation for the origin of HIV-2 in the cross species transmission of SIVsm from naturally infected sooty mangabey monkeys to humans.

Similarly, there is significant sequence homology between HIV-1 and a simian immunodeficiency virus, SIVcpz, isolated from a healthy chimpanzee.[11,12] Of note, chimpanzees experimentally infected with HIV-1 fail to develop overt disease despite establishment of infection as evidenced by transient viremia,[13-16] development of HIV-1 specific antibodies[17-19] and HIV-1 specific cytoxic T cells.[20-22] This constellation of observations have led to the widely held speculation that both human immunodeficiency viruses types 1 and 2 have evolved independently following cross-species transmission from a common group of lentiviruses of African primates.[10] It is further speculated that the disease potential may be enhanced in the newly infected host. Rhesus macaques have not been demonstrated to be infected with SIV in the wild; however, an isolate of SIV (SIVmac) originating from a captive macaque who shared housing facilities with sooty mangabeys has shown the same degree of sequence homology as between HIV-2 and SIVsm.[23,24] Of particular interest is the development of an immunodeficiency syndrome in this macaque and other experimentally infected macaques with SIVsm.[24] The clinical immunodeficiency syndrome which develops in these animals closely mimics the clinical features of HIV-1 infection.[24] Similarly, Cynomolgous monkeys, which also appear not to be infected in the wild, are quite susceptible to experimental infection with SIVsm and develop an immunodeficiency syndrome with a markedly compressed clinical course.[25] Finally, the unfortunate accident which led to a laboratory worker being infected with SIVsm may add further support for such cross-species transmission as the origin of the human immunodeficiency viruses.[26]

At the other end of the clinical spectrum, a recent isolate of SIVsm from an infected macaque has been shown to be rapidly fatal, usually leading to death within 5-14 days.[27-29] Molecular characterization of this viral isolate has failed to clearly establish the basis for its increased pathogenicity, although there are some significant sequence changes from the less pathogenic parental strain of SIVsm.[27] A similar, although less dramatic, disease variability has been observed with HIV-1 where there are reports of long term survivors for as many as 15 years[30-32] and recent estimates that at least a few patients will never develop disease (personal communication to Pomerantz); and reports of patients who rapidly progress to immunodeficiency in a matter of a few years.[33,34] Comparison of clinical courses between the two human HIV species suggest a significantly prolonged clinical course with HIV-2 infection when compared with HIV-1.[35]

This complex pattern of clinical expression among lentiviruses is shared by the other species of retroviruses to be considered herein. The human spumaviruses (or foamy viruses) have yet to be clearly associated with *any* disease in humans despite certain populations with a high prevalence of infections; and the ready culture of infectious virus in explanted tissue culture.[36,37] Among the complex oncoviruses, human T-cell leukemia/lymphoma virus type II (HTLV-II) has been shown to be endemic in certain Paleo-American Indians without clinical disease.[38] By contrast, infection with human T-cell leukemia/lymphoma virus type I (HTLV-I) in a minority of patients leads to either adult T-cell leukemia if acquired in infancy or a chronic neuropathic disease if acquired later in life.[38] Despite many similarities among these viruses, there are marked differences in the level of clinical expression; yet, it is apparent by the maintenance of infection within these populations that some level of infectious progeny virus is generated from these various integrated proviral sequences.

Despite the vast research effort on retroviruses in the last 10-15 years, there is still little known of the mechanism of disease production by these pathogens. It is unclear why SIVagm which has the same overall genomic organization as the other lentiviruses causes no known disease in its native host, the African green monkey. Similarly, it appears that SIVsm probably causes no significant disease in its natural host the sooty mangabey and yet causes an AIDS-like illness in experimentally infected rhesus macaques and cynomolgus monkeys. SIVsm may have been the origin of HIV-2 which causes one of the clinical AIDS syndromes in humans. While there are genomic differences between the rapidly fatal variant of SIVsm and other SIVsms, the differences fail to clearly define the pathogenic moiety of this virus.[27] Within the oncoviral family of complex retroviruses, HTLV-I when acquired in infancy in southeast Japan leads to ATLL in a small minority of people, while in the majority of people, it remains clinically latent throughout life.[38] In certain Caribbean populations, however, where infection is acquired later in life, infection with HTLV-I leads primarily to a neuropathic disease.[38] HTLV-II, in contrast, which is endemic in certain isolated populations throughout the world (and appears to be gaining a foothold in certain populations using intravenous drug) causes no known disease.[38] HIV-1, which has devastated certain human populations, is most closely related to SIVcpz which appears to cause no disease in either naturally infected or experimentally infected chimpanzees. What has become clear, however, is that the final disease potential of retroviruses lies in the complex interaction of the integrated provirus with the infected host. This interaction takes place in at least two major arenas: the immune system which struggles to eliminate virally infected cells, constantly challenged by mutation of neutralizing epitopes; and the host cell's transcriptional control of the integrated proviral genes. This book will examine the latter of these interactions, the determinants of proviral gene expression in the context of surrounding cellular genes. To accomplish this goal we will systematically review the regulatory sequences of selected retroviruses and the multiple potential cellular transcriptional factors which interact with these sequences. In addition, we will examine a number of virally derived transactivating proteins which impact on the overall level of viral gene expression. Finally, in light of the unique life cycle of these agents, we will discuss the emerging view that chromatin structure provides an additional level of transcriptional control over integrated proviral sequences.

HISTORY OF RETROVIRUSES

It has been over 80 years since the first description of an infectious agent that would ultimately be identified as a retrovirus. Equine infectious anemia virus (EIAV) was identified as the etiologic agent of episodic hemolytic anemia of horses in 1904.[39] Despite this early description, it would be 70 years before it would be assigned to the lentivirus subfamily of retroviruses.[40] A few years later, in 1911, Rous would describe another infectious agent that would give birth to the field of RNA tumor viruses. For nearly four years he visited a New York City market near Rockefeller University where he collected chickens with soft tissue tumors. During this time he collected over 60 spontaneous tumors of chickens.[41] Attempts to passage these tumors in other chickens was at first difficult, however, with each successive transfer, the tumors grew faster and metastasized to more sites. Finally, after several transfers, Rous was able to induce tumors simply by injecting filtered material from this tissue.[42] This agent, the Rous Sarcoma Virus, would decades later be identified as a member of another group of retrovirus, the oncoviruses.

Numerous other reports would soon follow of transmissible agents leading to tumor formation in animals. One of the more interesting of these agents is the mouse mammary tumor virus (MMTV) which continues to yield important insights into the retroviral-host cell interaction today and in retrospect demonstrated the concept of retroviral latency in its initial description. In the early 1930s in the genetics laboratory of Castle at Harvard University, inbred strains of mice were being developed. One of these strains (C3H) was developed for its high incidence of mammary tumor formation in the female offspring. A second strain was developed for its low incidence of tumor formation. From selective matings between the strains, it was shown that the high tumor phenotype developed only when the female partner of the mating was from the high incidence strain.[43] It was soon demonstrated that this high incidence of tumor formation in the female offspring of these animals could be largely eliminated by separating the newborn mice at birth and foster breastfeeding them by low tumor incidence females.[44,45] Further studies established a filterable agent in milk which was capable of imparting the high tumor incidence phenotype on the offspring of either the high incidence strain or the low incidence strain.[45,46] Of greater interest in terms of retroviral latency was the subsequent demonstration that the male offspring of the high incidence strain, while not spontaneously developing tumors, could be induced to form tumors by estrogen injections.[47,48] These observations suggested that merely carrying the genetic material of this agent was not sufficient for its phenotypic expression; from this data came the concept of a "latent infection." Only in the last decade have the molecular mechanisms of hormonal induction of latent MMTV been established in any detail (discussed in detail in chapter 3).

Parallel to the development of the field of oncoviruses was the less heralded but equally informative development of the field of lentiviruses. In 1933 several sheep of the Karakul breed were imported from Germany to Iceland to boost wool production. The sheep appeared healthy during the 2 months of quarantine prior to release into the native sheep population. However, from 1935 through 1951 three new diseases of the sheep population began to appear.[49] The first of these, visna, was identified in the southern districts of Iceland where sheep were developing a paralytic and wasting syndrome.[50,51] While the clinical presentation was variable, often presenting with subtle gait disturbances or failure to thrive, the infection invariably progressed to death over several months to years.[49] Pathologically, there was diffuse demyelination of white matter throughout the central nervous system.[49] Within the same geographic area a second new disease was also noted, pulmonary adenomatosis.[52] In the northern districts, Gislason identified yet another form of pulmonary disease, a chronic progressive pneumonia given the name "maedi," an Icelandic term for dyspnea.[53] It was not until the late 1950s that tissue culture techniques were available to grow the agents of these various diseases at which time it became apparent that they represented different manifestations of the same viral infection.[49,54] All of these diseases were epidemiologically linked to importation of the sheep from Germany. Of particular note was the long period from infection to development of disease, ranging from two to six years. This long clinically latent period gave rise to the designation of this class of viruses as lentivirus from the latin word "lenti" for slow. This group of viruses now contain a number of relatively newly described agents including human immunodeficiency virus type 1 (HIV-1), human immunodefeciency virus type 2 (HIV-2), simian immunodeficiency virus (SIV), feline immunodeficiency virus (FIV), Visna, bovine immunodeficiency virus (BIV), equine infectious anemia virus (EIAV) and caprine arthritis and encephalitis virus (CAEV).

A third group of retrovirus is the spumavirus or foamy virus. These agents were first identified as "contaminants" of monkey kidney cells adapted to tissue culture in the mid 1950s.[55] Their name derives from the cytopathic appearance of infected cells in tissue culture where the cytoplasm is filled with vacuoles, giving a foamy appearance.[36] In addition to a high prevalence of infection in monkey kidney explants, a number of serotypes of simian foamy virus (SFV) were identified in the quest to identify the agent of Kuru. Gajdusek isolated a number of strains of SFV from explants of chimpanzee brains (as well as many other tissues) with experimentally transmitted Kuru.[56] It would soon become clear that these viruses were not the etiology of Kuru but represented naturally occurring, clinically latent viral infections of monkeys that were reactivated upon explant culturing. The first *human* retrovirus isolated, also by explant culturing of tumor cells, was in fact, a "foamy virus" from a patient with nasopharyngeal carcinoma in 1971.[57] Given the apparent widespread infection of primates with these foamy viruses, an attempt was made in the 1970s to define the serologic prevalence of human infection with these agents. One seroprevalence study identified as high as 5% of certain human populations in Africa with evidence of infection.[58] Despite this high prevalence, there was no clearly identified illness associated with this infection just as there was no identified illness associated with non-human primate infection with SFV. In addition to primate infections, spumaviruses have been isolated from cats, bovine, rodent and sea lions.[37] Because of the lack of clinical disease associated with these infections, they were largely ignored until only recently.

By the 1970s the seminal discovery of Temin[59] and Baltimore[60] that RNA viruses could be reversed transcribed from RNA into DNA and subsequently integrate into the host cell's DNA changed the concept of viral pathogenesis and ultimately tied the oncoviruses, lentiviruses and spumaviruses into the family *Retroviradae*. With this fundamentally different life cycle it became possible to envision viral infection with this class of agent as chronic persistent infections rather than acute cytopathic (but self limited) infections. Despite these early descriptions of a number of animal retroviruses it was not until the 1980s that the first well documented human retrovirus was described that was convincingly associated with disease.[61] A stable T-lymphoblastic cell line called Hut 102 was established from a lymph node biopsy of a 28-year-old patient with a cutaneous T-cell lymphoma. Reminiscent of the experience of Rous where numerous passages in chickens were required to produce free virus, this cell line at first only produced viral particles after induction with 5-iodo-2'-deoxyuridine. After numerous passages, however, the cell line began to continuously produce virus with all of the features of an oncovirus.[61] A year later came the isolation of another virus from a 64-year-old patient with cutaneous manifestations of T-cell leukemia (Sezary syndrome)[62] which proved to be closely related to the first virus. These viruses were designated human T-cell lymphoma/leukemia virus (HTLV).[61,62] Within the next two years a second human retrovirus would be isolated which was sufficiently different to gain designation as human T-cell leukemia/lymphoma virus type II. This virus was isolated from a patient with the very rare T-cell variant of hairy cell leukemia.[63] Despite its isolation from this patient it became clear over the next few years that it was not the etiological agent of hairy cell leukemia. Indeed, (as discussed in chapter 4), it has been discovered to be endemic in certain populations throughout the world without any apparent disease association.[64,65]

At about this same time came the first clinical descriptions of an acquired immunodeficiency syndrome. In 1981, Gottlieb published the case reports of four homosexual men who developed *Pneumocystis carinii* pneumonia without any recognized underlying illness.[66] Laboratory evaluation revealed dramatically low CD4 (Leu3+) positive lymphocyte counts and elevated suppressor (Leu2+) to helper lymphocyte (Leu3+) ratios. While not fully appreciated at the time, this would prove to be the initial description of the AIDS epidemic in the United States and would bring recognition to a recently described wasting disease of Africa. Within the next 3-4 years there would be a flurry of reports linking this new clinical syndrome with a human retrovirus, ultimately designated human immunodeficiency virus type 1 (HIV-1).[67-74]

Not long after the initial studies of HIV-1, a second etiologic agent of the clinical syndrome of AIDS was described almost exclusively in West Africa, that of human immunodeficiency virus type 2 (HIV-2).[75] While these clinical syndromes shared many features, HIV-2 has remained largely confined to West Africa and appears to be a somewhat less virulent pathogen. The intense scrutiny of retroviruses resulting from the study of these new human pathogens, HIV-1 and HIV-2, has led to a greater appreciation of the widespread prevalence of retroviral infections throughout the animal kingdom; and no doubt many new disease associations will be established as the study of human retroviruses continues.

PHYLOGENY AND TAXONOMY OF RETROVIRUSES

One of the tasks of the retrovirologist today is to analyze the biological behavior and nucleotide sequence of newly described retroviruses and group them into functional and evolutionary units. These classifications not only aid in scientific communication but provide a framework from which to advance hypotheses about behavior based upon sequence, or predict sequence based upon biological behavior. The basic genomic organization of retroviruses led to an early attempt to divide retroviruses into two groups: the simple retroviruses and the complex retroviruses.[76] All retroviruses contain three essential genes termed gag, pol and env. In addition, they contain regulatory sequences in the two identical long terminal repeat (LTR) sequences located at the 5' and 3' ends of these structural genes. The simple retroviruses produce only these three basic components necessary for production of infectious viral particles. By contrast, the complex retroviruses contain a number of regulatory genes in addition to these three basic gene products.

There are a number of additional features of retroviruses that lend themselves to more discriminating classification schemes.[24,26] The most obvious feature of these agents is their ability to reverse transcribe single stranded RNA into double stranded DNA. The enzyme reverse transcriptase (RT) is a virally encoded protein whose genomic diversity has served as one basis for lineage assignment of many retroviruses.[25,27] Many such lineage trees have been generated either based on RT comparisons or comparison of other segments of the retroviral genome. Figure 1.1 shows a simplified lineage scheme of the retroviruses to be considered herein. This representation is not intended to reflect the precise degree of relatedness among these viruses, nor to represent all of the proposed seven genera of retroviruses, but rather to provide an overview of the relation of viruses under discussion. As discussed above, this phylogenetic tree clearly supports the view that the two human immunodeficiency viruses have evolved independently and share more sequence homology with their paired simian immunodeficiency virus than with each other. Similarly, the human T-cell leukemia viruses (HTLV I & II) share significant homology with each other and with the simian T-cell leukemia virus. Of interest, (just as with the human and simian immunodeficiency viruses), there is mounting evidence that many species of monkey are also infected with the simian counterpart of the HTLVs.[70] It will be of particular interest to watch the development of more detailed lineage maps of these complex onco-retroviruses to determine if (and when) the human viruses were acquired from non-human primates as the immunodeficiency viruses seem to have been. The isolation of HTLV II from certain geographically isolated

Indian populations suggests that this virus has been in humans for a relatively long time when compared to the acquisition of HIV.

While spumaviruses were the first retroviruses to be isolated from humans, they remain the stepchild of retrovirologists precisely because of their non-pathogenic nature. They are, in fact, a testament to the remarkable accommodation that can take place between retroviruses and their "sponsoring" host who appears to be relatively unharmed by their presence. The creation of finer lineage maps for the human and non-human primate spumaviruses will hopefully shed light on their origin and date their introduction into the human population.

RETROVIRAL LATENCY

The selected few retroviruses outlined in Figure 1.1 reflect a broad spectrum of clinical disease "penetrance" which has been the basis for the concept of retroviral latency. The term *latent* derives from the Latin for hidden. As molecular technology has advanced, however, the application of the term latent has become blurred. It has, for example, become clear that in the majority of cases of human spumavirus infection clinical disease is inapparent. This clinical latency may reflect cellular latency as well in that viremia with spumaviruses has not been routinely documented. By contrast, explant culturing of many tissues from spumavirus infected individuals can readily produce virus establishing the criteria, as defined for this discussion, of true latency; that is, there is a fully competent proviral genome present which is unexpressed at baseline but capable of re-activation. By contrast, infection of African green monkeys with SIVagm is clinically latent, yet there is ready isolation of infectious virus from these animals' circulation suggesting that at least some of the infected cells within this host are not latent at the cellular level. Similarly, HIV-1 infection leads to a clinically latent period lasting years, yet inevitably progresses to clinically apparent illness and ultimately death. Here too, there is ready isolation of virus from the circulation (with the appropriate techniques) throughout the clinically latent period. A closer look at the individual cellular level, however, demonstrates the majority of infected CD4+ cells to be latently infected, in that they contain integrated proviral sequences but fail to make functional transcripts (discussed in detail in chapter 2). To avoid the historically ambiguous use of the term latent, we will consider retroviral gene expression not as an "all or none" event but rather in terms of the relative levels of restriction to viral gene expression at the individual cellular level.

In the overview provided above, it is apparent that the host-retrovirus interaction is complex; and the complexity of this interaction arises, at least in part, from the unique life cycle of these viruses. The phylogenetic relationships among the various groups of retroviruses to be discussed herein also appear to segregate along this spectrum of clinical disease. The human and simian immunodeficiency viruses represented in the upper portion of Figure 1.1 appear to be the most virulent pathogens (at least in humans) where there is nearly 100% penetrance of disease. One of the central mysteries of the pathogenesis of AIDS is the near uniform illness that follows infection of humans with HIV-1;

and yet in the chimpanzee, where HIV-1 (or SIVcpz) likely arose, infection fails to produce any disease in either the natively infected animals or experimentally infected animals. Chapter 2 is devoted to an detailed examination of the large body of data on the transcriptional control mechanisms of HIV-1. These data are then compared with the limited data available on transcriptional control of SIVcpz as discussed in chapter 4.

While it is too early to conclude that HIV-2 will have a lower disease penetrance, at least at this point in the AIDS epidemic, the

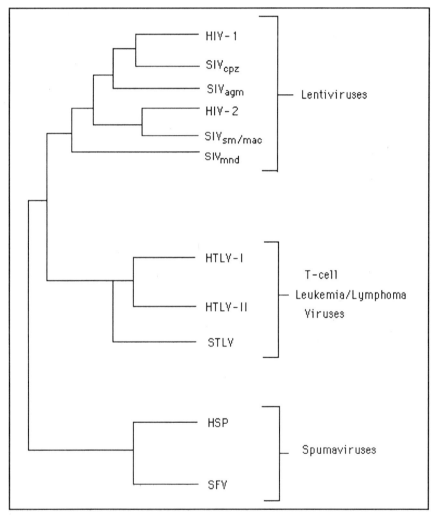

Fig. 1.1. A simplified lineage scheme of retroviruses. This phylogenetic tree is not intended to quantitatively represent evolutionary distances between viruses but to illustrate the relative relatedness between these infectious agents. As can be seen, there is a greater sequence homology between HIV-1 and SIVcpz, and between HIV-2 and SIVsm/mac, than there is between the two human pathogens HIV-1 and HIV-2. Also of note in this phylogenetic tree is the obvious parallel between infection of human and non-human primates. For each class of human pathogen represented, there is a closely related simian retrovirus.

clinical course appears to be more prolonged. In an attempt to determine the reason for such a difference we will consider in chapter 4 the transcriptional control mechanisms of HIV-2 and those of various SIVs. While these delineations are somewhat arbitrary in that many of the SIVs are more distantly related to each other than they are to the HIVs, direct comparisons will be made to HIV-1 where possible with a particular emphasis on the role of the host plays in disease production.

The complex primate onco-retroviruses (HTLV I & II, STLV) shown in the middle portion of Figure 1.1 represent a somewhat greater potential for clinical latency. As will be discussed in chapter 4, only a minority of humans (or non-human primates) will eventually express clinical disease despite a near life-long infection with this group of retroviruses. Spumaviruses, shown in the lower portion of Figure 1.1 and also discussed in chapter 4, represent the opposite end of the spectrum in terms of retroviral latency. Despite nearly two decades of searching, there is no clearly associated clinical illness with either the human or non-human primate infections. Finally, in chapter 3 retroviral latency will be considered in the context of the infected host. Given the unique life cycle of retroviruses, any consideration of proviral gene expression must take into consideration the effect of the random integration event and how the individual cell "manages" its newly acquired retroviral gene cluster.

CHAPTER 2

HUMAN IMMUNODEFICIENCY VIRUS TYPE 1

Current estimates of the number of HIV-1 infected people in the world stands at 10-12 million.[78] In well developed countries, where there is ready access to health care, the clinical face of HIV-1 is changing. In the initial stages of the epidemic in the United States, most patients died of *pneumocystis carinii pneumonia* (PCP). As the medical community became more effective at treatment and prophylaxis of PCP, it became clear that other opportunistic infections merely replaced PCP as a cause of death. It was no mystery that these opportunistic infections reflected the immunosuppression that resulted from a dramatically reduced CD4+ lymphocyte count. What remained a mystery, however, was how HIV-1 led to this CD4+ lymphocyte depletion/dysfunction.[79,80] A number of hypotheses were advanced, including infection with co-pathogens,[81] stimulation of a superantigen,[82] HIV-1 induced programmed cell death (apoptosis),[83] dysfunctional cell surface signaling[84] and even a very small contingent which questioned whether HIV-1 infection was, in fact, the cause of AIDS.[85] Central to this debate was the apparent low level of HIV-1 infection of CD4+ cells in peripheral blood mononuclear cells (PBMCs), the relatively low level of circulating virus early in disease, and the long incubation period from infection to clinical disease. Consequently, a great deal of effort has been devoted to determining the sequence of events which follow the initial infection with HIV-1 and how these events might lead to such profound immunosuppression. Figure 2.2 briefly reviews the life cycle of HIV-1 in the infected CD4+ lymphocyte. While we will concentrate on the life cycle of HIV-1 in the CD4+ lymphocyte, it is clear that other host cells are involved in the pathogenesis of HIV-1 infection (such as monocytes/macrophages, neurons, astroglia, B-lymphocytes and dendritic cells)[86] and may selectively influence certain portions of this viral life cycle.

EVIDENCE THAT HIV-1 LATENCY EXISTS AT THE CELLULAR LEVEL

Following acute infection with HIV-1, there is a high level of plasma viremia, lasting days to weeks.[98-99] This is followed by a prolonged period, lasting years, during which there is minimal detectable virus

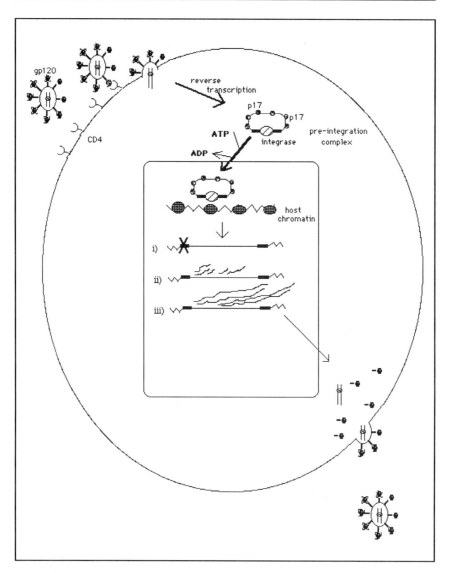

Fig. 2.2. The high affinity interaction of the surface glycoprotein of HIV-1 (gp120) with the CD4 molecule of the helper T lymphocyte leads to the subsequent fusion of the viral particle (perhaps with the help of the hydrophobic portion of gp41) with the cellular membrane. This allows entry of the HIV-1 core where there is completion of reverse transcription of the viral genomic RNA and simultaneous formation of a pre-integration complex.[87,88] This complex is moved through the nuclear membrane by an energy requiring process into the cell's nucleus[89] where there is integration of the proviral DNA into the host's genome. Unlike simple retroviruses, HIV-1's (and probably all lentiviruses') pre-integration complex can be transported into the nucleus independent of cell division.[90,91] On a macroscopic scale, integration is a random event, although recent data suggest that local chromatin configuration creates favorable integration sites[92-97] and the site of integration may subsequently influence the pattern of proviral gene expression (see chapter37). Once integration takes place, there are three basic patterns of proviral gene expression that can occur: (i) complete latency where there is no initiation of transcription; (ii) transcriptional initiation which generates either non-processive or multiply-spliced messages that fails to generate progeny virus; and (iii) full length transcripts which are effectively orchestrated to generate HIV-1 structural gene products as well as accessory and regulatory gene products (tat and rev) with production of progeny virus.

in the circulation.[100,101] Recent evidence implicates the generation of HIV-1 specific cytotoxic T cells as critical to the initial control of plasma viremia.[102-104] In many respects, the initial phase of HIV-1 infection parallels that of other acute viral infections. What sets it apart from other infections however, is the persistence of proviral sequences within its target despite this immune response. It has been these observations that raise the question of the level of transcriptional activity of the integrated provirus during this clinically asymptomatic stage of infection with HIV-1. One mechanism whereby an infected cell could elude immune destruction is by maintaining its proviral sequences transcriptionally silent. Indeed, by in situ hybridization for HIV-1-specific transcripts, there are estimates of only 1 in 10,000 to 1 in 100,000 peripheral blood mononuclear cells (PBMCs) expressing detectable levels of proviral-derived messenger RNA.[105] By contrast, the number of PBMCs estimated to carry HIV-1 proviral sequences determined by quantitative polymerase chain reaction (PCR) has ranged from approximately 1 in 100 to 1 in 1000 during the early asymptomatic stages of infection[106-109] and even higher during the end stages of disease.[110,111] Approaching this issue from another perspective, Bagnarelli et al recently attempted to determine the mean transcriptional activity of infected PBMCs by quantitating plasma virion RNA in relation to circulating proviral copy number per defined quantity of cells. They demonstrated that for the majority of patients in the asymptomatic stages of disease, this ratio was less than 1.[112] This evidence strongly suggested that the vast majority of cells carrying proviral sequences were not actively expressing viral transcripts in vivo. The limitation to this technique of DNA end-point dilution PCR, however, is that it fails to distinguish viral burden at the single cell level as in situ RNA hybridization does; it therefore remained formally possible that all infected cells actively expressed viral transcripts but that each infected cell carried multiple copies of HIV-1 provirus accounting for this discrepancy.

To better define this level of viral burden, more sensitive techniques were needed to resolve infection at the single cell level. This was accomplished by in situ DNA PCR.[113-117] Bagasra et al showed by this technique that even in early stages of disease, there were nearly 1% of PBMCs that carried HIV-1 proviral sequences;[113] and with advancing disease that percentage reaches as high as 40-60% of CD4+ cells.[114] Embretson et al similarly showed by in situ DNA PCR of a tumor biopsy from an HIV-1 infected individual that approximately 15% of the infiltrating mononuclear cells (lymphocytes and monocytes) had detectable proviral sequences. By contrast, with in situ RNA hybridization of the same tissue, there were less than 1 in 1000 mononuclear cells that were actively expressing HIV-1 specific transcripts;[114] this suggests that greater than 99% of infected mononuclear cells failed to express detectable levels of viral RNA. They and others have recently extended these findings to lymphoid tissue from patients at various stages of disease.[115,118,119] Finally, Patterson et al have shown with in situ PCR followed by hybridization with a fluorescinated probe that they could subsequently sort cells based on the amplified proviral DNA product.[120] They too demonstrate a significantly higher number of

PBMCs carrying proviral DNA than are actively expressing HIV-1 specific transcripts.[120] These data support the proposal that at a cellular level the majority of cells infected with HIV-1 are latently infected, in that they express no detectable levels of viral RNA by standard methods.

What has not been definitively established, however, is whether these cells fulfill the definition of viral latency in that they carry a replication competent provirus in a quiescent form rather than simply a defective provirus. Restricted viral expression in a number of chronically infected cell lines have been demonstrated to be inducible including the TE671/RD,[121] U1,[122,123] OM10,[124] J1.1[124] and ACH2[125] cells, demonstrating that certain cellular clones can indeed carry a replication competent HIV-1 provirus in a relatively quiescent form. What has also become clear from these studies is that more than one mechanism of restriction to viral expression is at play.[124,126] In U1 cells, there appears to be a restriction imposed by the cellular milieu, whereas in ACH-2 cells, the block to viral expression appears to be mediated by the site of integration.[127-129] Several laboratories have demonstrated that ACH-2 cells, when superinfected, fully support high levels of viral replication but only of the superinfecting virus and not of the original infecting virus. Despite this, the native virus is fully infectious and grows normally when transferred to another cell.[127-129] By contrast, U1 cells fail to support high levels of replication of either the native or superinfecting virus and appear to have an abnormal nuclear factor *kappa* B (NF-κB) family of transcriptional factors to account for the restricted level of expression.[130]

Recent studies have begun to address activation of virus production from lymphocytes of HIV-1-infected patients[131-133] rather than from these immortalized CD4+ cell lines. Preliminary evidence suggests that primary lymphocytes from HIV-1-infected patients can be induced to produce high levels of virus by several cell surface signaling pathways.[131-133] One such mechanism involves stimulation of primary lymphocytes isolated from HIV-1 infected patients with soluble anti-CD3. CD3 is involved in antigen specific T-cell proliferation by association with the T-cell receptor. Interestingly, phorbol myristate acetate (PMA) or phytohemmaglutinin (PHA) by themselves were very poor inducers of p24 antigen from primary PBMCs, both of which are potent inducers of HIV-1 production in lymphoid and monocytoid cellular model systems of latency.[122,123,125] By contrast, stimulation with immobilized anti-CD3 had significantly less of an effect despite its marked effect on stimulation of cellular proliferation.[133] It has further been shown that this effect of soluble anti-CD3 requires T-lymphocyte-monocyte interaction.[132] If either the receptor-counter-receptor pair of CD2:LFA-3 or CD18:ICAM-1 is blocked by monoclonal antibodies, this effect of soluble anti-CD3 is significantly dampened.[132] These data would suggest that: (i) there may be a difference in the reactivation mechanism between primary mononuclear cells infected in vivo and immortalized CD4+ cell lines infected in vitro; (ii) that the signaling pathway requires a cell surface interaction between T-lymphocytes and monocytes; and (iii) that reactivation of latent proviral expression is not merely a function of cellular proliferation. This effect of anti-CD3 can be further augmented by cross-ligation with anti-CD28[131], a surface receptor on CD4+ cells that mediates increased expression of nuclear factor-kappa B (NF-κB) and interleukin-2 α.[134]

Given the central role of the CD4+ lymphocyte in the pathogenesis of HIV-1 disease, it is not surprising that the majority of attention has been devoted to this population of cell. Another significant participant, however, is the monocyte/macrophage.[135-138] In other lentivirus infections, the macrophage has been proposed as a "Trojan horse" where it serves as the vehicle for wide dissemination of infection;[139,140] and may well serve this function in HIV-1. It is the most frequently infected cell identified in solid tissue such as brain, skin and lymph nodes.[141-146] Circulating monocytes have also been demonstrated to be infected, with the vast majority being latently infected.[147-151] Mikovits et al demonstrated the highly restricted nature of monocyte infection in vivo.[147] They isolated and purified monocytes from a number of asymptomatic seropositive patients. At a level of detection of 1 proviral copy in 100,000 cells they were able to detect HIV-1 DNA in only 9 of 21 patients' monocyte cultures. When co-cultures with Con-A activated T cells however, they were able to recover fully infectious virus from 90% of patients indicating the presence of at least one latently infected cell within the monocyte culture. In addition, they demonstrated that a CD4 positive cell line (HUT 102) could not substitute for activated T lymphocytes in this rescue of virus. Furthermore, they demonstrated that cell-cell contact was required for rescue and that partially purified membranes from activated T cell could activate virus production from these monocytes.[147] Schrier et al extended these observations and attempted to more fully define the requirements for T cell mediated activation of viral expression from monocytes infected in vivo.[150-151] Through a series of experiments they demonstrated that cell contact was required between the T cell and monocyte for the first 24 hours of incubation, that the lymphocyte involved in this interaction was of the CD4+/CD8- phenotype, and that this induction could be blocked by antibody to LFA-1 or IL-1 but not to IL-2. Furthermore, activation protocols which did not employ antigen presentation by the monocyte/macrophages failed to rescue virus from these cultures.[150] These observations suggested that cellular membrane contact during early events in the activation process of T cells was critical to differentiation and reactivation of HIV-1 from latently infected monocytes. It has been further suggested that differentiation of monocyte/macrophages prior to HIV-1 infection in vitro also affect the level of viral production. In vivo derived terminally differentiated cells such as alveolar macrophages or in vitro differentiated monocytes support greater viral production than non-differentiated peripheral monocytes.[149] While the molecular details involved with monocyte/macrophage differentiation by activated T cells are very sparse, it is potentially significant that the initiation of an antigen specific immune response in vivo involves direct T-lymphocyte-monocyte/macrophage interaction and may provide the necessary format for eliciting HIV-1 production from latently infected tissue macrophages or may facilitate the direct cell to cell spread of HIV-1 from macrophage to CD4+ T cell.

Another question remaining is whether the low but detectable levels of circulating virus in plasma is in fact from a small percentage of these latently-infected cells that have subsequently reactivated HIV-1 proviral expression or whether it derives from a hidden sanctuary of cells that are continuously expressing virus which subsequently finds access to the circulation. Indeed, the findings of Embretson et al with in situ PCR of the tumor tissue where fewer than 0.1% of mononuclear cells infected with HIV-1 were expressing HIV-1 viral transcripts, surprisingly revealed that the tumor cells themselves (derived from an adenocarcinoma of the lung) had a high level of proviral sequences and were expressing dramatically high levels of HIV-1 specific transcripts.[114] It is tempting to implicate the participation of cellular tumor suppressor genes, such as p53, in this high level HIV-1 gene expression (see below). Pantaleo et al have similarly reported a significantly higher level of HIV-1 viral RNA in lymph nodes, as compared to circulating PBMCs of HIV-1-infected individuals.[119] While these findings have been supported in other laboratories, it appears that this high level of viral RNA represents trapped viral particles in the interstices of lymph nodes rather than a high level of local proviral transcription[115,152] and the actual number of virion particles in the germinal centers of lymph nodes have been estimated to be on the order of 10^9 particle per cubic millimeter.[153] The clinical significance of these apparently antibody coated, trapped virions within lymph nodes remains to be determined. Another noteworthy finding of the study of lymphoid tissue compared with circulating PBMCs is the relatively higher percentage of cells which carry the provirus by in situ DNA PCR (at least in the early stages of disease) and the higher percentage of cells which yield virus upon coculture.[115,118,119] Finally, two recent studies have compared sequences from virion RNA from plasma compared with sequences derived from proviral DNA in circulating lymphocytes; and both studies suggest that the template from which the circulating virion RNA is derived is not from circulating lymphocytes.[154,155] In light of the recently demonstrated importance of the generation of HIV-1 specific cytotoxic T lymphocytes (CTL) in the initial control of infection, the unexpressed proviral templates in these circulating PBMCs may reflect the cellular survival advantage that results from maintaining their provirus transcriptionally silent.[102,103]

While it remains to be determined whether the circulating levels of virus in the asymptomatic stages of HIV-1 infection are the result of reactivation of previously quiescent provirus in circulating mononuclear cells, or whether circulating virus originates from another population of tissue-associated cells (such as lymphoid tissue) that are continuously replicating virus, it is clear that a majority of the circulating mononuclear cells, infected early in HIV-1 infection, do not produce detectable levels of virus.[115] It would also preliminarily appear that these T-lymphocytes and monocyte/macrophages are capable of reactivation in vitro[131-133,147-151] and therefore fulfill the narrow criteria for latency as considered herein. It is our opinion that the current debate over the existence of HIV-1 latency is largely a semantic one. There is clearly clinical latency in that there is no apparent disease for many years following the initial infection. Similarly, at an individual cellular level there iare very compelling data to support proviral latency in the vast majority of cells at any given time. On an organismal level, however, there are small but detectable levels of circulating virus throughout the course of infection with HIV-1 and therefore cannot be considered to be a truly latent infection on an organismal level. This low level viremia during the clinically latent period likely stems from a small minority of productively infected cells which have either escaped immune elimination or from latently infected cells which have reactivated viral production in response to an environmental stimulus.

ELEMENTS OF VIRAL GENOME STRUCTURE CONTRIBUTING TO VIRAL GENE EXPRESSION

Any attempt to delineate the mechanisms involved in establishing latency in these infected circulating mononuclear cells requires evaluation of both the HIV-1 virus's input to its transcriptional control as well as the cell's input. A brief overview of the genomic organization of the integrated provirus and the potential gene products and their function is required.[156-158] Figure 2.3 shows the overall genomic organization of HIV-1 with the flanking cellular genomic DNA. The full length viral transcript serves as both the genomic RNA for assembly into virions and the template for translation of the Gag and Pol polyproteins. These polyproteins are subsequently cleaved into smaller proteins with various functions. The 55 Kd Gag gene product is cleaved into p24, p17, p9 and p6. The p24 protein is the core structural antigen of the virus; p17 is a matrix protein and has recently been identified as part of the large pre-integration complex which is actively transported to the nucleus of the infected cell;[159] p9 contains a Cis/ His motif and participates in virion packaging by interaction with the ψ site; and the function of p6 remains to be fully established. The Pol polyprotein is cleaved into the reverse transcriptase enzyme, the integrase enzyme, and the protease enzyme. The Env gene is a singly-spliced transcript which is translated into gp160; this protein product is subsequently cleaved to form the two virally determined components of the outer membrane of the virus, gp120 and gp41. These proteins mediate attachment and entry of virus into cells.[156-158]

In addition to these basic gene products which are common to all retroviruses, HIV-1 has a number of additional regulatory proteins which contribute significantly to its overall complexity. These proteins result from translation of multiply-spliced mRNA species. Two of these products, *tat* and *rev*, are central to the overall level of expression of viral transcripts and of the splicing pattern of these transcripts and thereby bear directly on the level of HIV-1 viral production. The exact contribution of the singly-spliced accessory genes *vpu*, *vif* and *vpr* to HIV-1's level of transcriptional activity remains to be determined. They probably contribute more to the assembly and transport into and out of cells than to a determination of transcriptional activity and will not be further discussed herein. We will examine three major aspects of the molecular control of HIV-1 transcription: (i) the mechanism of *tat* transactivation; (ii) the role of *rev* in control of splicing patterns of

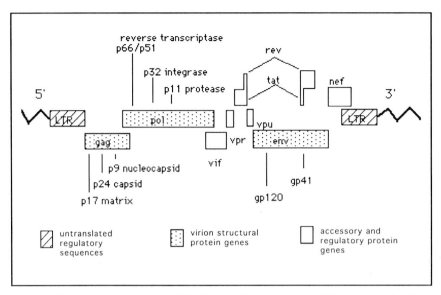

Fig. 2.3. Genomic organization of HIV-1. Like all retroviruses, HIV-1 contains the three structural genes: gag, pol, and env. Each of these yield a polyprotein which is subsequently cleaved (either by a cellular enzyme or viral enzyme) into functional viral constituents. Also like all retroviruses, HIV-1 contains identical repeats flanking the structural genes, the long terminal repeats (LTR). Unlike the simple retroviruses, however, HIV-1 contains a number of other gene products which result from differential splice site usage. Two of these gene products, tat and rev, significantly impact on the level of viral replication. The impact of the other gene products (vif, vpr, vpu and nef) are still being determined.

viral transcripts; and (iii) the multiple potential interactions of cellular transcriptional factors with the HIV-1 LTR.

Tat

The HIV-1 viral *tat* protein is the product of a multiply-spliced mRNA yielding an 86 amino acid protein. This viral gene product is an essential regulatory protein for the efficient replication of the virus. Much has been learned about its mechanism of action and it has defined a new class of "transcriptional" factor, which includes those that function through RNA rather than DNA. The transactivating potential of this viral gene product was initially appreciated by the dramatic "*trans*"-activation of HIV-1 LTR-dependent reporter constructs, where 50- to 300-fold stimulations were observed in the presence of *tat* protein.[160-163] The essential target region within the viral LTR was soon defined by mutational analysis and shown to reside *downstream* of the transcriptional start site (Fig. 2.9 and 2.10).[163-165] This region, the transactivation response element or TAR, is located from approximately +14 to +45 relative to the transcriptional start site.[166,167] This TAR sequence was shown to be orientation and position dependent with loss of *tat* function if moved from its immediate downstream position or placed in an opposite orientation.[168-171] These unusual properties of the *tat*/TAR interaction were an early clue to the unique nature of this viral gene product.

Since the TAR element was located downstream of the transcriptional start site, it could act either through DNA or RNA. The TAR region RNA was predicted to have an extended stem-loop structure[169,172] which was subsequently shown to be important for transactivation.[173-177] The elegant studies of Berkhout et al took an important first step in precisely defining the interaction of *tat* with its target RNA.[178] They designed experiments where the stem-loop structure of the RNA was altered without altering the precise base pair sequence of either the RNA or DNA within the TAR region. They introduced antisense sequences into the RNA *outside* of the defined TAR element which would, however, modify the secondary structure assumed by the RNA and showed the critical nature of the "bulge" in the ascending arm of the stem-loop structure.[178] This trinucleotide bulge has subsequently been shown to be the binding site for *tat* and its formation essential for *tat* function.[179-184] Furthermore, they showed through this same strategy that this structure needed to be present in the nascent RNA as it was being transcribed for *tat* to function.[178] Analysis of the TAR stem-loop structure also identified another critical feature, the hexanucleotide loop, which was required for *tat* transactivation in vivo.[185-187] It is widely held that this structure binds a host cell specific factor since no direct binding of *tat* to the loop has been demonstrated. In addition, a number of reports describing such a factor(s) have recently appeared.[188-195]

The importance of this loop was further demonstrated by the use of "TAR decoys" in a attempt to prevent *tat* transactivation. Sullenger et al showed that overproduction of TAR RNA elements from an independent promoter dramatically reduced the level of native HIV-1 viral production within an infected cell.[196] This inhibition was generally assumed to result from competition between the "decoy" TAR RNA elements and the native TAR RNA elements transcribed from the infecting virus.[196] Extension of these studies did, indeed, demonstrate the requirement of the *tat* binding bulge in the stem of the decoys to achieve inhibition of viral production. Surprisingly, however, it was also demonstrated that the loop structure was required to achieve inhibition.[197] These latter findings argue against the simple notion that the "decoy" TAR elements were "absorbing" the available *tat* preventing it from interacting with the native TAR sequences.[197] These findings rather support the earlier observations that both the trinucleotide bulge and the hexanucleotide loop are required for *tat* transactivation; and may suggest that there is a transactivating protein complex which forms over the stem-loop structure consisting of both the viral specific *tat* protein and a cellular specified loop binding protein. One potential explanation for the requirement of both elements for inhibition of viral production by the "decoy" TAR structures is that the cellular protein may stabilize the contact of *tat* with a very short RNA target and without this stabilization the competition for *tat* binding favors the native TAR elements produced from the infecting virus.[197] In fact, it had been long suggested that one reason rodent cells do not support high levels of HIV-1 expression is the lack of this loop binding protein (which maps to human chromosome 12).[198,199]

While both the *tat* binding bulge and the loop structure of the
TAR element seem to be required for *tat* transactivation in the native
setting of the HIV-1 LTR, it is interesting that other heterologous
RNA targets can substitute for the TAR element. The coat binding
protein of bacteriophage MS2 is a sequence specific RNA binding protein.
Selby and Peterlin demonstrated that replacing the TAR element of
HIV-1 (maintaining the appropriate spatial positioning relative to the
LTR) with the RNA target for coat binding protein still led to
transactivation by *tat* if the *tat* protein was fused to the binding domain of the coat binding protein.[200] Similarly it was shown that the
rev response element (RRE), (the sequence specific RNA target of the
HIV-1 *rev* protein) could substitute for the TAR element in achieving
tat transactivation if fused to the binding domain of *rev*.[201,202] Finally,
the block to high level expression of HIV-1 LTR-driven genes in ro-
dents could be overcome by using the *tat*-MS2 coat binding fusion
product targeted to the coat binding specific RNA element.[203]

In summary, *tat* transactivation of the HIV-1 LTR requires the
highly structured TAR element which has two essential components,
the direct *tat* binding trinucleotide bulge and the hexanucleotide loop
structure. This loop structure in all likelihood binds a specific (human) cellular protein(s) which may stabilize the *tat*/TAR interaction
that ultimately results in transactivation.

While it is clear that the *tat* protein leads to increased viral gene
expression it is less clear whether *tat* functions to increase transcriptional initiation, to improve transcriptional elongation, or to increase

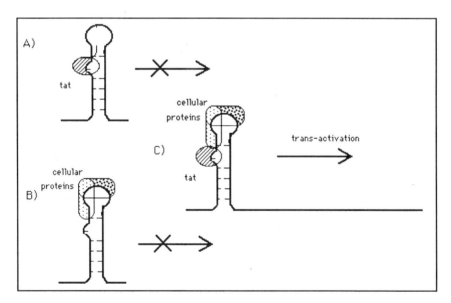

Fig. 2.4. The TAR RNA forms a highly stable secondary "stem-loop" structure that results
in a trinucleotide "bulge" in the ascending arm of the stem as well as a hexanucleotide
"loop" at the apex of the stem. The trinucleotide bulge is the target for Tat binding,
however, (A) Tat binding alone is insufficient for transactivation. Similarly, (B) binding of
the loop specific cellular factor(s) is insufficient for transactivation. Only in the presence
of both elements (C) of this protein:protein:RNA complex does efficient up-regulation of
steady state HIV-1 specific mRNA occur.

translational efficiency. The preponderance of data on the transactivating potential of *tat* clearly demonstrate that its principle action is to increase the steady state levels of HIV-1 specific RNA.[204-206] What remains of some debate, however, is the relative contribution of increased transcriptional initiation versus improved transcriptional elongation to this overall up-regulation of steady state RNA. Early assumptions were that *tat* functioned primarily by increasing transcriptional elongation since it bound to RNA rather than DNA as do most traditional transcriptional factors.[207] Indeed, there is a body of evidence to support a primary role for improved transcriptional elongation as the mechanism of *tat*'s transactivation. Kao et al reported in transient expression assays that in the absence of *tat*, greater than 85% of correctly initiated transcripts failed to elongate past the first 55-60 base pairs.[168] By contrast, in the presence of *tat* greater than 99% of transcripts fully elongated. In addition, there was an approximate 50-fold increase in the overall expression of the LTR driven transcripts. Because the short transcripts were found in the cytoplasm[173] it was concluded that they did not simply represent pausing of the RNA polymerase but premature termination of transcripts and therefore concluded that *tat* acted as an anti-terminator.[168] It would be predicted that if there was a specific termination signal within the first 55-60 base pair (overcome in the presence of *tat*) that deletion of this region would have a similar effect, that is to promote full length transcripts. This was in fact shown *not* to be the case.[207] Other data suggested that rather than a specific termination at position 59 within the HIV-1 LTR, there was random termination throughout the length of transcription. Comparison of transactivation between *tat* and E1A proved to be insightful. Laspia et al showed that there were essentially two classes of transcripts originating from the HIV-1 transcriptional start site: (i) short transcripts of variable length and (ii) full length transcripts.[208] In comparing the transactivating effects of the well characterized adenovirus E1A protein and *tat*, it was demonstrated that *tat* increased only the level of full length transcripts whereas E1A increased both the long and short transcripts. In addition, E1A and *tat* were found to act synergistically.[209] This data suggested that E1A acted to simply increase the rate of transcriptional initiation without effecting the polarity of transcripts. By contrast, *tat* effected primarily the polarity of the transcripts; that is, more of the initiated transcripts were fully elongated.[208] This divergence of effect was further supported by the synergy demonstrated between these two transactivating proteins,[209] one increasing the rate of initiation (E1A) and the other increasing the proportion of the initiated transcripts which reached full length (*tat*).[208] These observations led to the proposal that *tat* acted as an RNA processivity factor.[173] Two studies of in vitro transcription from the HIV-1 LTR did in fact, demonstrate such an effect. Marciniak and Sharp demonstrated two classes of elongation complexes by in vitro transcription from cell free HeLa nuclei: one leading to transcripts of less than 500 base pairs and another leading to full length transcripts.[210] Using discontinuous probes to define transcript lengths, they demonstrated that in the absence of *tat* only 2% of transcripts that reached position 82 proceeded through position 1495. Once transcripts reached greater than a 1000 base pairs however, there was a much greater likelihood that the transcripts would reach full length. These observations strongly suggested that rather than a uniform population of elongation complexes (which would not be predicted to give a biphasic response) there are two classes of elongation complexes, one processive and one not.[210] In the presence of *tat* however, there was an increase in the percentage of initiated transcripts that fully elongated. By the same token, if *tat* merely contributed to the processivity of each complex of a uniform population of elongation complexes then there should not be a polarity to the *tat* effect. In fact, the transacting effect of *tat* was seen predominantly in the transcripts of less than 800 base pair with little effect on transcripts of greater length. This again argued for two elongation complexes with two inherently different processivity potentials and that the presence of *tat* increased the percentage of the more processive complexes. Quantitative estimates of this population of processive complexes in the absence and presence of *tat* were 10% and 50% respectively.[210] Of interest in this in vitro system, there was no apparent increase in the rate of transcriptional *initiation* in the presence of *tat*.[210] Similarly, Lu et al demonstrated two different classes of transcriptional complexes in vivo through a series of fine mutations created within the HIV-1 LTR.[211] They found that Sp-1 and NF-κB sites generated processive complexes in the absence of the TATA box whereas in the presence of the TATA box both classes of complexes could be formed. More significantly, the formation of non-processive complexes required the TATA box, and only the non-processive complexes could be transactivated by *tat*.[211]

Independently reported data provided by Berkhout and Jeang demonstrated that the minimal requirement for a basal level of expression from the HIV-1 promoter was contained within nucleotide positions -43 to +80.[212] Although this segment of the genome contains the TAR sequences, this minimal promoter was not *tat* responsive. To achieve *tat* inducibility they needed to add some form of upstream enhancer such as NF-κB (the most efficient), Sp-1, AP1 or Oct. They too show a marked preference for the HIV-1 TATA sequences for *tat* inducibility.[212] There is in fact some evidence of direct binding between *tat* and Sp-1 and to a lesser extent between *tat* and NF-κB (see below and ref. 273).

Finally, placement of sequences that tightly bind cellular factors 3' to the TATA box prevented efficient elongation.[211] This short stretch of DNA from -5 through +59 has been named the inducer of short transcripts (IST) by several authors.[213,214] While this model teleologically would appear to be inefficient (continuous generation of short, non-processive transcripts) there is precedent for such a transcriptional system. The heat shock transcriptional complex in *Drosophila melanogaster* behaves similarly.[215] The RNA polymerase II transcriptional machinery is continuously engaged and proceeds a short distance downstream where there is termination. In the presence of the induced heat shock protein there is rapid relief of the downstream obstruction and procession to full length transcripts. In the case of heat shock protein there is evidence that the obstruction is from a precisely positioned nucleosome which upon induction of heat shock protein is displaced (or at least modified).[215] It is postulated that genes which require a very rapid response time to external signals are maintained in this posture despite the high energy requirements. It is unclear why a cell would maintain the HIV-1 genome in a "rapid response" mode. There is, however, at least preliminary data to suggest that under certain circumstances it does. In the U1 cell line which is maintained in a very restricted state of viral production, there is evidence of abundant promoter-proximal transcripts[216] which can be converted to predominantly promoter-distal transcripts by providing *tat* alone, either as purified protein or as a *tat* expressing plasmid.[128,216] Of even greater interest is the similar finding in PBMCs from asymptomatic seropositive patients where only promoter-proximal transcripts could be detected.[216] This is in contrast to late stage disease where full length transcripts (spliced and unspliced) predominate. These observations would suggest that even in some latently infected cells there is a significant level of transcriptional initiation that occurs but which fails to elongate in the absence of *tat*. It should be noted however, that in another model of cellular latency, the ACH-2 cell line, *tat* alone fails to significantly effect the level of proviral transcription,[126,128] which again, underscores the potential for multiple mechanisms of proviral latency.

Similar results on elongational processivity were observed by Kato et al who extended these findings to show that *tat* may interact with cellular transcription factors or partially substitute for them.[217] It has been suggested that the cellular transcription factors TFIIF and TFIIS both function to increase elongation efficiency.[218-221] These authors demonstrated that (under the specialized in vitro transcription system utilized) *tat* dramatically increased transcriptional elongation as previously shown; however, this increased elongational efficiency could also be achieved with purified TFIIF and obviate the need for *tat*. By contrast, TFIIS acted synergistically with *tat*. Finally, antibody to the large subunit of TFIIF appeared to preferentially suppress *trans*-activation by *tat* in this transcription system.[217] The simplest model to accommodate these observations is that *tat* functions by recruiting or stabilizing the entire RNA polymerase II complex (perhaps through a physical interaction with TFIIF) leading to improved elongational efficiency.

In parallel with the development of the model of *tat* functioning to enhance elongational efficiency, there was somewhat contradictory data accumulating to suggest that *tat* could function as a traditional DNA binding transcriptional factor if provided the necessary targeting domain. Kamine et al and Southgate and Green independently demonstrated that *tat,* when fused with the DNA binding domain of the GAL4 transcription factor, could mediate *trans*-activation just as native *tat* does in the presence of TAR if the cognate sequences for GAL4 binding were placed immediately upstream of the Sp-1 sequences.[222,223] In addition, the Sp-1 sequences were required for the *tat trans*-activation. This data would suggest that *tat*, in fact, functions as a traditional DNA binding transcriptional factor with the exception that its targeting mechanism is through the nascent RNA stem loop structure rather than DNA sequences. In addition to the above mentioned E1A transactivation (a prototypic acidic transactivator) VP-16 was shown by some laboratories to be functionally equivalent to *tat* when targeted to the nascent RNA derived from the HIV-1 LTR; that is, it could accomplish its transactivation by binding to an already initiated transcript.[202] By contrast, however, if VP-16 and *tat* are compared in their ability to transactivate heterologous promoters when targeted to DNA binding sites, *tat* remains Sp-1 dependent while VP16 is not.[224] Similarly, through a series of fusion proteins, Ghosh et al showed that while VP16 and *tat* could both transactivate reporter genes when targeted to upstream DNA, that VP16 was much more efficient in doing so.[225] In addition, the effects of VP16 targeted to DNA and *tat* targeted to RNA were shown to be synergistic suggesting that the precise

Fig. 2.5. (A) Despite the presence of the TAR element with this minimal transcriptional unit containing only the TATA and initiator elements, this construct is poorly responsive to tat *and generates non-processive, short transcripts. (B) Similarly, in the presence of Sp-1 sites and NF-κB sites but without an HIV-1 TATA box, these transcripts remain poorly responsive to* tat, *presumably as a result of the generation of highly processive transcripts which do not benefit from the tat/transcriptional machinery interaction. (C) In the presence of all of the basic core promoter/enhancer elements, there are two transcriptional complexes generated, I and II. Complex II is processive and non-*tat *responsive while complex I is non-processive and* tat *responsive. The precise structural differences between complex I and II remain to be defined but probably reflect the overall stability of the assembled proteins at the TATA element. Interestingly, both complexes remain responsive to the adenovirus transcriptional trans-activator E1A which directly binds the general transcriptional factor TFIID; however, the relative number of transcripts to reach full length remain constant in the presence of E1A suggesting a fundamentally different mechanism of action between this transactivator and* tat.

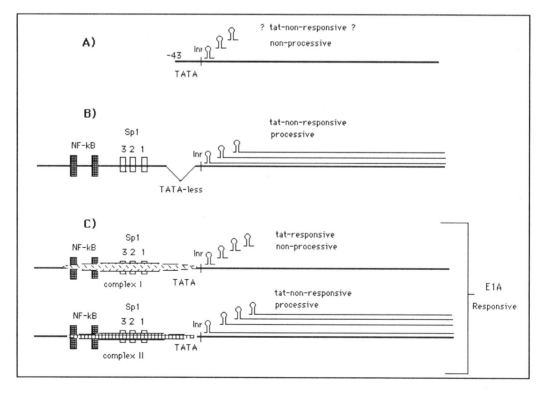

mechanism of transcriptional activation differed.[225] Also of note is the greater efficiency of *tat* transactivation when using the HIV-1 TATA box rather than a heterologous TATA box.[212,226] These data suggest something unique to the assembly of the transcriptional complex on the HIV-1 promoter with respect to its interaction with *tat*.[224,226] An attempt to determine if the rate limiting step in transactivation by *tat* is this complex assemblage of proteins or release of some downstream pausing event led to a unique set of experiments.[227] Jeang and Berkhout engineered self-cleaving ribozymes just downstream of the TAR element such that it would not effect the TAR secondary structure but would separate (upon cleavage) the *tat*:TAR complex from the remainder of the elongating RNA complex. With a rapid cleaving ribozyme, there was abrogation of the *trans*-activating effect of *tat*. They could however restore *tat*'s function by replacing the rapid cleaving ribozyme with a slow cleaving ribozyme in the same position.[227] They conclude from this data that the rate limiting step in *tat*'s transactivation is the completion of the *tat*:TAR:LTR interaction and not a downstream event.

Finally, in support of *tat*'s function as a more traditional DNA transcriptional factor, there are several recent reports of TAR independent *tat trans*-activation of the HIV-1 LTR, again suggesting that *tat* has some primary effect upon the viral promoter.[228-232] It should be pointed out that this TAR independent *tat trans*-activation appears to occur under specialized circumstances such as in the background of central nervous system derived cells[228,230,231] or in the presence of potently stimulated nuclear factor-kappa B (NF-κB).[229,230] Whether such events will contribute significantly to the overall level of circulating virus remains to be determined.

While the above data does not firmly establish the mechanism of *tat* transactivation, one model proposed to accommodate most of the accumulated information is that there are two inherently different transcriptional complexes assembled on the HIV-1 promoter: one processive and unresponsive to *tat* and the other non-processive but responsive to *tat*.[233] The non-processive complex is strictly dependent upon the presence of the HIV-1 TATA box and upstream Sp-1 sites. By contrast, the processive complex can form in the absence of the TATA box and is more efficiently assembled under the influence of the NF-κB:enhancer interaction (see below). Under baseline conditions, the majority of complexes fail to elongate and transactivators such as E1A (which merely increase transcriptional initiation) lead to an increase in full length transcripts but preservation of the ratio of non-processive to processive complexes (with the vast majority being non-processive). In contrast, *tat* leads to an increase in the ratio of processive to non-processive transcripts and, perhaps, an increase in initiation of transcription. While the role of the TAR sequences at first appeared to be unique to *tat*'s function, it now appears to be merely a targeting sequence for the positioning of *tat* (along with a cellular-TAR RNA loop binding protein(s)) to the HIV-1 promoter. Finally, the *tat*:transcriptional complex interaction which results in a more elongationally competent complex may involve direct contact with the general transcription factor TFIIF.

Using an HIV-1 LTR driving the human interleukin-2 gene, Cullen demonstrated an increased ratio of interleukin-2 protein to interleukin-2 mRNA in the presence of *tat* suggesting that in addition to increasing the steady state level of LTR driven mRNA, *tat* also increased translational efficiency.[165] Similar results were suggested by a number of other laboratories who demonstrated that a portion of the *tat* effect was evidenced post-transcriptionally.[234-239] Other data however refute a significant translational effect of *tat*[240] and at present the predominance of data support *tat*'s major contribution to HIV-1 viral gene expression at the level of transcriptional control.

Tat Protein

Mutational analysis of the *tat* protein has demonstrated a number of functional domains within the first exon.[241-249] The three major domains identified by most authors consist of: (i) the acidic N-terminal region which is the transactivating region of the protein; (ii) the cysteine rich region containing seven highly conserved cysteine residues; and (iii) the basic domain which serves to localize the *tat* molecule to the nucleus and provide the actual binding site for TAR. The C-terminal end of the molecule contributed largely by the second exon appears (at least in transient transfection assays) to be largely dispensible.[243,247,248,250] Initial studies which identified the N-terminal region as the transactivation domain utilized fusion proteins with various targeting sequences borrowed from DNA binding proteins.[200,201,222,223,251] It was demonstrated that the first 48 amino acids of this N-terminal region were sufficient for transactivation if provided with the necessary DNA binding realms. This acidic region is predicted to form an amphipathic α-helix and will tolerate a few conservative amino acid substitutions if they maintain the overall helical structure.[252] It is tempting to speculate that the mechanism of *tat* transactivation is similar to other well characterized DNA binding transcriptional factors with acidic activation domains which share this helical conformation. In fact, recent evidence suggests that the first 48 amino acids of *tat*, when fused to the GAL4 DNA binding domain (without the GAL4 activating domain), can transactivate the GAL1 promoter.[253] This would suggest the helical, acidic activation domain of *tat* may indeed function in a "generic" fashion similar to other acidic activation domains. It remains to be proven, however, whether these initial observations are of functional significance in the *tat* transactivation of the HIV-1 LTR.

The cysteine rich domain is highly conserved among complex retroviral *tat* proteins;[254,255] and as might be predicted is intolerant of substitutions of the cysteine residues (with the possible exception of cysteine 4).[242,243,248,249] It is predicted that this region binds divalent cations; is the site for homodimer formation (although the formation of homodimers in vivo has yet to be proven); and contributes to the overall secondary structure of the protein.[246]

The third functional region of the *tat* protein is the basic domain. This short stretch of nine highly basic amino acids contains a nuclear localizing sequence and is the actual binding site of *tat* to TAR.[179-183,256,257] It appears that *tat* binds to the first uridine residue (U23) in the bulge of the TAR RNA stem.[258,259] In addition, from extensive mutagenesis studies by Churcher et al, the two residues (G26 and A27) immediately downstream of the bulge (formed by the U23,C24,U25 residues) along with their corresponding base pairs (C39 and U38); and the two residues immediately upstream of the bulge (A22 and G21) along with base pairs (U40 and C41) also contribute to the strength of *tat* binding to TAR RNA.[259] Studies of short synthetic peptides of *tat* however, suggest that there is some additional contribution of the N-terminal domain to the specificity of *tat* binding.[260]

The C-terminal portion of the *tat* protein which is encoded within the second exon of the *tat* gene has been shown in transient transfection assays to be largely dispensable for its function.[243,247,248,250] Whether the same can be said for natural infection where the target for *tat*'s function originates from an integrated HIV-1 provirus has recently been questioned. Jeang et al have recently demonstrated that both exons of *tat* are required for maximal *tat* transactivation from an integrated LTR whereas only the first exon was required for efficient transactivation from an unintegrated LTR.[261] These findings are interesting in light of an earlier study showing *tat*'s function to be influenced by the site of integration. Kessler and Mathews showed by nuclear run-on assays that *tat* functioned to increase both transcriptional initiation as well as elongation in the setting of low basal levels of transcription and this basal level of transcription was determined by the position of adjacent sequences such as the SV40 promoter.[262] Under conditions of high basal expression, *tat* appeared to function only to increase elongational efficiency without an effect on the already high level of transcriptional initiation. The *tat* construct used in these studies contain both exons of *tat*.[262] One potential explanation for these findings is that the second exon of *tat* functions to overcome the inherently low level of basal expression of integrated plasmids by increasing transcriptional initiation. Under transient transfection conditions, the basal level of expression is above the threshold at which the transcriptional initiating function of *tat* is significant and therefore the second exon is dispensable. This would offer an explanation for the continued usage of the second exon in natural infections where the target of *tat*'s function is the integrated provirus whose basal level of transcriptional initiation might be expected to be low. This proposal might also offer insight into the debate as to whether *tat* functions to increase initiation in addition to improving elongational efficiency; that is, under experimental conditions leading to low basal, *tat* accomplishes both functions while under experimental conditions leading to high basal expression only the elongational function is apparent.

Additional synthetic peptide studies have yielded some intriguing results, the significance of which remain to be determined. Vives et al made a series of synthetic *tat* peptides including full length *tat* protein.[263] They report that peptides containing residues 1-48 fails to *trans*-activate an LTR driven reporter construct which is not surprising in the absence of a targeting sequence contained in the basic domain (in contrast to Jeyapaul et al[264]). Similarly, they report that peptide 38-60 which contains the basic domain for TAR binding and nuclear local-

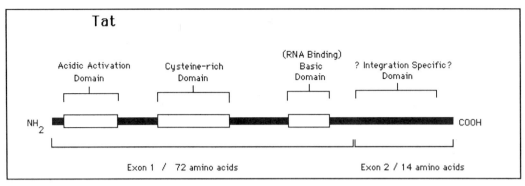

Fig. 2.6. Linear representation of tat with its functional domains. While generated from two exons, most investigators find the second exon of tat dispensable for transactivation of the HIV-1 LTR. The acidic activation domain shares some features with other acidic transactivating transcriptional factors; however, it is not established that these similarities translate into shared mechanism(s) of activation. The basic domain provides nuclear localization as well as the specific binding site for the trinucleotide bulge of TAR RNA. The cysteine rich region probably provides some 3-dimensional structural stability necessary for tat function. While there is still some debate as to the function (or significance) of the second exon of tat, it is of note that in natural infections the majority of tat appears to be derived from both exons suggesting some in vivo utility.

ization but not the N-terminal region fails to transactivate (similar to Frankel et al,[141] but in contrast to Green and Lowenstein[265]). Unexpectedly, however, when these two peptides were used together, there was significant transactivation of the HIV-1 LTR despite these two domains being expressed on separate peptides.[263] It is hard to imagine, in the absence of the unlikely event that there is a direct affinity between these two peptides, how providing the binding domain and the transactivating domain on separate moieties could achieve transactivation within the model proposed; that is, TAR RNA functioning as a target for binding of *tat* whose transactivating domain is then positioned to interact with the assembled transcription factors on the LTR. Similarly puzzling data exist on *trans*-dominant negative mutants of *tat* which contain a mutation in the basic domain.[266,267] It would be predicted that these mutant proteins (with a non-functional basic domain) should have no effect on *tat*'s ability to transactivate since they fail to bind TAR RNA. Some of the explanations advanced for such an effect is the formation of inactive heterodimers between the functional *tat* and mutant *tat* proteins.[166] Arguing against such an explanation is the lack of data to suggest that dimerization between *tat* molecules even occurs in vivo. Another explanation offered is the binding and sequestration of cellular *tat* binding proteins which appear to be essential for *tat*'s transactivating potential.[166] It has generally been accepted that these cellular proteins interact with the loop structure of TAR rather having a primary interaction with *tat* as would be required of this latter explanation. Despite the great attention devoted to this novel protein, it is apparent that *tat* has resisted a simple, straight forward dissection of its mechanism of action. Nevertheless, *tat* remains a critical determinant of proviral gene expression and will remain an important target of therapeutic strategies.

TAT: TAR AND THE CELLULAR PROTEIN "CONNECTIONS"

The initial observations that murine cells failed to support high level *tat* transactivation proved both frustrating and enlightening.[198,199] While eliminating a traditionally useful collection of cell lines and animal models for the study of *tat*, it led to the identification of a number of cellular proteins which interact with *tat* and TAR. One cellular protein identified from HeLa extracts is TRP-185 which is a 185 kilodalton protein shown in gel electromobility shift assays to bind with high affinity to TAR RNA.[166,188,265] TRP-185 shows a number of interesting binding specificities. It fails to bind to RNAs with base substitutions within the loop; while it bound in the presence of mutations within the bulge of the stem, if RNA was constructed and the distance between the bulge and the loop of the stem was increased, binding was abrogated.[166,188] In some assay systems it can transactivate the HIV-1 LTR in the absence of *tat*[268] and in other systems it is dependent upon *tat* for TAR-mediated transactivation.[188] It is of note that in sedimentation assays, that TRP-185 appears to be complexed to at least one other cellular protein which remains to be fully characterized.[166] In keeping with the many mysteries of *tat* function, while TRP-185 appears to be required for effective *tat* mediated transactivation and appears to bind the loop region of TAR RNA (unaffected by bulge mutations) it appears to *compete* with *tat* for TAR RNA binding.[166,268] One trivial explanation is that the assay system of gel electromobility shifting utilized in these experiments is not a true representation of in vivo three-dimensional structure and that in vivo the close approximation of these two molecules on non-overlapping regions of the TAR RNA leads to a more stable association for both. In any event, TRP-185 appears to be important for TAR mediated *tat* transactivation.

A second RNA binding protein has recently been identified.[268] This protein, TRP-2, surprisingly binds the bulge region of TAR RNA and like *tat* is dependent upon the first uridine residue within the bulge. Even more surprising, rather than inhibiting *tat* function by direct competition for TAR RNA binding, there is a minimal enhancing activity associated with its presence with *tat*.[268] Several other poorly characterized proteins have been reported to bind the stem-loop region of TAR RNA. One is a 68 kilodalton protein isolated from HeLa extracts which binds to the loop sequences.[189,269,270] Two additional cellular proteins which have been shown to recognize a portion of the double stranded stem structure are P1/dsI and SBP.[271,272] The significance of these potential TAR RNA:protein interactions remains to be determined.

In addition to TAR RNA binding cellular proteins, there are *tat* binding proteins. Two of these proteins have been mentioned above. On *tat* affinity columns, Sp-1 has been shown to be a direct *tat* binding protein which has obvious significance in terms of *tat*'s transcriptional potential.[273] Also discussed above is the direct binding of *tat* to the transcription factor TFIIF. This binding may have further significance in explaining the apparent interaction of cellular protein kinase C (PKC) with *tat* transactivation (beyond PKC's effect on the NF-κB:IkB dissociation).[274,275] *Tat* itself does not become phosphorylated but the

RAP30/74 subunit of TFIIF does.[276,277] It is interesting that 5,6-dichloro-1-β-D-ribofuranosylbenzimidazole (DRB) which is a compound that selectively inhibits cellular elongation factors such as TFIIF (and *preferentially* inhibits *tat* transactivation compared with basal transcriptional activity) is proposed to function by interfering with a cellular kinase activity.[210]

Nelbock et al described a cDNA derived from screening a λgt11 library whose 404 amino acid protein, designated TBP-1, binds *tat*.[278] Through a series of fusion protein constructions combining the TBP-1 protein with DNA targeting sequences from other proteins, TBP-1 was shown itself to have transcriptional activity with certain promoters such as HIV and thymidine kinase (TK).[279] In contrast, it failed to activate other promoters such as MMTV. Furthermore, mutations within either the purported helicase domain or within a nucleotide binding domain of the TBP-1 protein abrogated transactivation.[279] Two other closely related proteins have been identified which share 42-49% amino acid homology with TBP-1.[280,281] One of these, MSS-1, was isolated from a HeLa cell cDNA library and its level of expression within cells has been correlated with *tat*'s transactivation potential.[280] In P19 cells where there was little endogenous MSS-1 expression, co-transfection with an MSS-1 expressing plasmid markedly increased *tat*'s transactivation. In Jurkat cells however, where there are high levels of endogenous MSS-1 expression, co-transfection of this plasmid had essentially no effect.[280] In a somewhat more complicated series of experiments, Swaffield et al have identified a yeast protein, SUG1, which also shares significant amino acid homology with TBP-1 and is able to substitute for the GAL4 acidic transactivation domain in regulation of the yeast GAL genes.[281] These related proteins have been proposed as a new family of transcriptional factors which have at least some element of promoter specificity.[279]

In summary, *tat*'s transactivational effect is primarily reflected in increased steady state levels of HIV-1 specific mRNA. While the precise transactivational mechanism has not been defined, it would appear that *tat* binds TAR RNA resulting in the positioning of it (along with the essential associated cellular proteins), in close proximity to the assembling pre-initiation complex on the TATA element. This positioning may result in physical contact between *tat* and these transcriptional factors (such as TFIIF), or between the cellular proteins that accompany the *tat*:TAR complex. The apparent result of this close association is the conversion of a poorly functional pre-initiation complex (i.e. one that is non-processive) to a highly functional pre-initiation complex (i.e. one that is processive). As more fully discussed below, there is a developing theme in transcriptional regulation that the stability of the protein:protein:DNA complex at the transcriptional start site determines rate and efficiency of transcription. In light of this theme, one could speculate that the HIV-1 TATA element (which is important to *tat* responsiveness), lends itself to assembly of relatively unstable pre-initiation complexes, or complexes which are inefficient at displacing downstream obstructions. This might leave the HIV-1 provirus transcriptionally "poised" awaiting the arrival of the final component (the protein:*tat*:TAR complex) that will cement this mass of assembled proteins into a stable, functional unit that leads to production of full length mRNA. As our skill at in vitro transcription with purified transcriptional factors improves, it will hopefully be possible to define the exact *tat*:TAR interaction with the transcriptional machinery.

Rev

Rev is a 116 amino acid protein derived from a multiply-spliced mRNA which shares significant coding sequences with *tat*.[282,283] Like *tat*, *rev* is a unique RNA binding protein without known precedent in eukaryotic transcriptional systems. The splicing pattern of the complex retroviruses including that of HIV-1 make the maximal usage of the coding information contained within their genomes by using segments of the genome multiple times, in different combinations; as a consequence they must provide a mechanism for control of splicing patterns. There are four recognized splice donor sites and at least six splice acceptor sites within the HIV-1 genome which allows for a large number of potential mRNAs by differential usage of these sites.[283-289] In the eukaryotic nucleus, pre-mRNA is synthesized and, prior to transport to the cytoplasm for translation, undergoes removal of intronic sequences.[290,291] One of the impediments that HIV-1 must overcome for production of progeny virus is transport of its multiple species of mRNA to the cytoplasm, many of which contain intronic sequences. The initial description of a protein which would ultimately be shown to accomplish this function followed analysis of several mutants in the region downstream of the *tat* coding sequences.[292-294] These mutants failed to make progeny virus (or HIV-1 structural proteins) and yet contained transcriptionally active proviruses. Of note, however, was the overwhelming predominance of the multiply-spliced, 2.0 kb message. Differential examination of mRNA from the nuclear compartment compared with the cytoplasmic compartment revealed that there was normal production of all species of mRNA in the nucleus, with a selective loss of unspliced or singly spliced species in the cytoplasm in these mutants.[295-297] It was further demonstrated that this abnormal pattern of cytoplasmic mRNA expression could be overcome, in *trans*, by transfection of plasmids expressing the *rev* protein.[298,299] It was not long before mutational analysis of the HIV-1 genome identified the cis-acting element responsible for *rev* responsiveness.[297,300,301] This approximately 240 base pair region located in the intronic region between the second and third exons of *tat*/*rev* (and within the env open reading frame) proved to generate a highly structured RNA element.[302,303] It was subsequently shown to be position independent but orientation dependent for its function;[297] and *rev* was further shown, like *tat*, to be a direct RNA binding protein.[304-309] The predicted structure of the RRE is schematically represented in Figure 2.7. The overall two dimensional structure forms a primary stem loop (SLI) from which there forms four secondary stem loop structures (SLII-SLV). While this extended stretch of RNA defines the *rev* responsive element (RRE), mutational analysis has demonstrated that with the exception of stem-loop II, much of the remainder of the RRE is dispensable for *rev* binding in vitro and *rev* responsiveness in vivo.[301,306,307,310-313] Within stem-loop

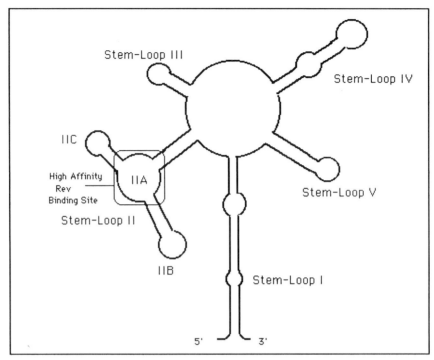

Fig. 2.7. Two-dimensional representation of the highly structured Rev Response Element (RRE). The RRE assumes a highly stable secondary structure consisting of the primary stem-loop represented as "Stem-Loop I." From this are generated four additional stem-loops numbered II-V. Stem-Loop II forms the primary site of rev binding with the high affinity site being generated by a 13 nucleotide "bubble" depicted by "Stem-Loop IIA."

II there is a 13 nucleotide sequence which has proven to be the sequence specific binding site for *rev* and involves a "bubble" that is stabilized by non-Watson-Crick base pairing within this bulge in the secondary RNA structure.[314] While the secondary structure of the RRE is important, *rev* binding is truly sequence specific. Dayton et al have shown in a series of constructs that generate the same secondary RNA structure as the native RRE but with different primary sequence, *rev* fails to either bind in vitro or function in vivo in the absence of the wild type primary sequence within stem-loop II.[315]

Unlike *tat*, *rev*'s binding has proven to be somewhat more complicated in that it requires oligmerization for its function. In addition, there appears to be several binding sites of differing affinity. Stem-loop II, alone, appears to accommodate three *rev* molecules.[305,316] The high affinity site within stem-loop II is defined by a 29 nucleotide sequence with the low affinity sites flanking it.[317] It is likely that the protein-protein interactions which take place (during oligmerization) after the initial binding of one molecule of *rev* to the high affinity site helps stabilize and strengthen the interactions with the low affinity sites (perhaps in conjunction with cellular proteins—see below);[318,319] although there is still some debate as to whether the oligmerization occurs prior to *rev* binding or whether this protein:protein interaction takes place after an individual molecule of *rev* binds to a high affinity site.[320,321] Regardless, *rev*'s maximal function occurs after the assembly of six to eight molecules onto the complex RRE structure.

Despite the significant information on the structural elements of the *rev*:RRE interaction, there is still not a firm understanding of exactly how *rev* accomplishes its function of allowing unspliced and singly spliced mRNA to escape the nucleus for cytoplasmic translation. One clue to the function of *rev* has been gained by tracking the travels of the *rev* protein within the various cellular compartments.[322-324] It has been established that *rev* shuttles back and forth between the nucleus (particularly the nucleolus) and the cellular cytoplasm and that preventing nuclear transport of cytoplasmic *rev* protein abrogates *rev* function. These findings are not surprising in light of its proposed function of safely escorting unspliced RNA out of the nucleus into the cytoplasm where it can undergo translation into HIV-1 structural proteins and serve as genomic RNA for viral assembly.

In an attempt to determine if the RRE could function within other cellular post-transcriptional regulatory pathways, Chang and Sharp placed the HIV-1 RRE in an intronic region of the β-globin gene.[325] Unexpectedly, *rev* was unable to substantially alter the splicing pattern of this gene unless the splice donor and acceptor sites of the β-globin gene were altered to make them less efficient. If the β-globin gene splicing signal was replaced by those of HIV-1 or the globin sites were mutated to create less efficient sites, *rev* could then serve to "rescue" intron-containing mRNA from splicing.[325] This would imply some competition between the splicing apparatus and the *rev*:RRE interaction; that is, with a very efficient splicing signal, the *rev*:RRE interaction loses the race to completion of splicing while in the presence of inefficient splicing signals, the *rev*:RRE interaction is able to compete with the splicing apparatus. In this light, it is interesting that Staffa and Cochrane have recently demonstrated the inefficient splicing of the *tat/rev* intron; and further demonstrated the splicing defect to be within the branchpoint region of the 3' splice site. Replacement of this 3' site with the efficient β-globin splice site resulted in high efficiency splicing.[326] It may well be that the inefficient splicing demonstrated by HIV-1 and other lentiviruses is critical to their remaining *rev* responsive by shifting the competition between the spliceosome and the *rev*:RRE complex in favor of the latter and thereby providing further flexibility for processing retroviral mRNA. While this model has some appeal, two recent studies to address this issue have yielded conflicting results. Hammarskjold et al provide data that the env mRNA of HIV-1 can be efficiently exported from the nucleus if the 5' splice site is removed and therefore not defined as an intron.[327] In direct conflict, however, Nasioulas et al show that elements other that splice sites determine retention of *env* mRNA within the nucleus in the absence of *rev*.[328] Yet another scenario has been proposed by Malim and Cullen, where rather than competition between the splicing machinery and the *rev*:RRE complex, there is a competition with other cellular factors which "mark" mRNA for degradation.[329] In either case, the remarkably complicated mechanism of pre-mRNA processing lends itself to a spectrum of perturbations favoring one outcome over another and it is likely that the *rev*:RRE interaction is one such perturbation favoring the survival of intron-containing HIV-1 specific mRNA.

Another potential, but less well characterized, mechanism of *rev* function is by displacement of inhibitory cellular factors from the poorly defined RNA sequences termed cis-acting repressive sequences (CRSs).[295,300,324,330-332] These ill-defined sequences, located outside of the RRE, appear to inhibit expression of HIV-1 mRNA's when present but can be overcome in the presence of *rev*. Exactly how *rev* might displace such putative factors remains to be determined. Other data support an improved association of the *rev*:RRE complex with cytoplasmic polysomes leading to improved translational efficiency.[333-335] While this may contribute in some measure to greater progeny virus production, it is clear that the major effect of the *rev*:RRE interaction is to increase the level of unspliced mRNA which escapes the nucleus.

Rev Protein

Like *tat*, *rev* is a modular protein. The N-terminal portion of the *rev* protein contains at least three identifiable (and physically overlapping) functions: (i) the RNA binding site, (ii) the oligomerization site and (iii) the nuclear localization signal; and the C terminal end provides the activation domain. The RNA binding site was initially defined by mutagenesis studies with in vitro binding assays. Amino acids 35-51 are the residues required for specific binding and 10 of these 16 residues are arginines.[336-338] This provides a highly charged region which is speculated to interact avidly with the phosphodiester backbone of RNA.[339] In addition, a synthetic peptide corresponding to this region was shown to bind specifically with the RRE.[305]

As discussed above, *rev* function requires multimerization. Even in the absence of an RRE substrate, *rev* in solution tends to form oligomers both in vitro and in vivo.[320,321,337,338,340-342] Mutagenesis studies have identified the short amino acid residues immediately flanking the arginine-rich RNA binding regions as the sites required for oligomerization.[316,336-338] While two early studies suggested that disruption of the multimerization sites prevented RRE binding,[337,338] a number of more recent studies suggest otherwise.[305,316,319,320,336,343,344] In addition, Daly et al and Madore et al have independently shown that the C-terminus of the *rev* protein is also involved in the oligomerization process.[319,345] While the precise three dimensional model of *rev* binding and multimerization remains to be defined, some of the data would suggest that the *rev* molecule binds as a monomer (through its basic domain and unaffected by the short oligomerization regions) to a high affinity site in stem-loop II of the RRE. This initial binding leads to attraction of additional *rev* molecules which bind to lower affinity sites but whose binding is stabilized by *rev:rev* interactions; and that this accumulation of additional *rev* molecules through interaction of these oligomerization residues is essential to *rev* function.

Also critical to *rev* function is its nuclear/nucleolar targeting sequences. This hexapeptide, Asn-Arg-Arg-Arg-Arg-Trp, located from residue 40-45 is essential for nuclear translocation of the *rev* molecule; and is essential for *rev* function.[303,323,346-349] Because this sequence overlaps

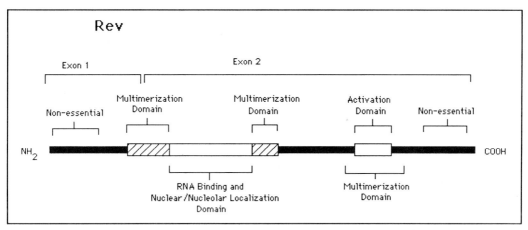

Fig. 2.8. Linear representation of the rev molecule with its functional domains. Rev is derived from two exons generating a 116 amino acid protein. There is a functionally overlapping domain near the amino terminus which provides nuclear/nucleolar localization in addition to RRE binding. Flanking this region are sites important to multimerization (and therefore function) of rev molecules. There is, in addition, a relatively poorly defined region near the carboxy terminal end of the molecule which also contributes to the multimerization function. Within this same region is the activation domain. The extremes of the amino terminal and carboxy terminal regions are dispensible to rev's function.

the RNA binding sequences it is not entirely clear if loss of function with mutation of these residues results from loss of RNA binding or loss of the nuclear localizing signal. In fact, *rev*'s relatively small size may allow free diffusion through the nuclear membrane; and, in fact, when this sequence is mutated, there is equal distribution throughout the cellular compartments without specific exclusion from the nucleus.[346,348,350] Similarly, it was initially felt that nucleolar localization was also essential to *rev*'s function; however, if RNA binding is maintained in the absence of nucleolar targeting, *rev* is still functional.[351]

A short leucine-rich sequence in the C-terminal portion of the molecule (residues 74-84) has been termed the activation or effector domain. Mutagenesis analysis has demonstrated that alterations within this region do not effect any of the other functions of the N-terminal region (with the possible exception of a contribution to oligomerization[319,345]) and yet completely abrogate *rev* function.[336,346,348,350,352-355] Since these mutations do not prevent nuclear localization or RRE binding, it has been suggested that they interact with some cellular factor(s) involved with splicing and/or degradation of mRNA. In support of such an effect, mutants in the activation domain act as *trans*-dominant negative inhibitors of *rev* function.[310,342,350,355-357] One hypothesis is that these mutants, which maintain their RRE binding ability, occupy sites that would otherwise be occupied by wild type *rev* molecules; and by doing so prevent the "normal" interaction of the *rev* activation domain with a cellular factor required for *rev* function. Curiously, a recent study shows that these *trans*-dominant negative mutants fail to multimerize in vivo.[318] One potential explanation for this finding is that the proposed cellular factor(s) which interacts with the activation domain of wild type *rev* can no longer stabilize this protein:protein association for lack of a functional C-terminal domain.[318] Alternatively, this finding may support the recent reports of Madore et al and Daly et al that the C-terminus is involved with oligomerization in addition to the short sequences flanking the basic domain.[319,345] Finally, some insight may be gained by the recent demonstrations that the functional domains of several other lentiviruses can substitute for that of HIV-1 in *rev's trans*-activation, despite the obvious lack of sequence homology.[354,358-360] What these activation domains have in common is a high leucine and proline content and a relatively hydrophobic character. It is difficult to determine if this basic motif is sufficient for *rev's* function in the absence of a clearer understanding of the precise mechanism whereby *rev* transports intron containing mRNA safely from the nucleus.

REV:RRE AND CELLULAR CO-FACTORS

True to the recurring theme of multi-protein participation in most cellular processes, *rev's* commandeering of unspliced mRNA from the cellular nucleus appears to involve other cellular proteins. As with *tat*, *rev* was found to be poorly functional in murine cells. Trono and Baltimore showed that the pattern of HIV-1 expression in a number of murine cell lines to be reminiscent of *rev* negative mutant viruses.[361] The wild type expression could be recovered with fusion of the murine cell lines with uninfected human cell lines leading to the obvious conclusion that, as with *tat*, a human derived cellular factor was involved in *rev's trans*-regulation.[361] While less straightforward, Ahmed et al proposed a similar hypothesis to explain the *trans*-dominant inhibition of *rex* (*rev's* counterpart in HTLV-1) or *rev* on their respective targets by a mutant of the other *trans*-regulatory protein; that is, a *rex* mutant could serve as a *trans*-dominant inhibitor of *rev's* function when bound to the HIV-1 RRE.[362] Similarly, a *rev* mutant could inhibit the function of *rex* when targeted to its RNA binding site.[362] While a number of possible explanations exist, one clear potential scenario was the interference of the wild type protein's interaction with a cellular factor (since there was no interference with either RNA binding or multimerization). It was not long after these reports in fact that a cellular protein was identified from a HeLa cell extract that bound *rev*.[363] Fankhauser et al identified a 38 kilodalton protein, B23, which bound specifically to *rev* immobilized onto an affinity column. Interestingly, B23 could be displaced from *rev* by the addition of HIV-1 RRE sequences but not by unrelated RNA.[363] It is of particular significance that B23 had been previously demonstrated to serve as a shuttle protein between the nucleus and cytoplasm for ribosomal elements.[364] These findings led to the proposal that B23 imports *rev* to the nucleus where it binds RRE containing sequences and is then transported to the cytoplasm with intron containing mRNA in tow as a complex with B23. If this model is accurate, it would suggest that nuclear localization is provided by B23 rather than the nuclear localizing sequences contained within *rev*. As discussed above, because these sequences are so intimately involved with RRE binding, it will be difficult to separate these functions. Additional cellular proteins have also been nominated for participation in *rev*'s function by the demonstration of their binding specifically to the HIV-1 RRE RNA.[365,366] One of these proteins is a 56 kilodalton protein derived from HeLa extracts which multimerizes in the presence of RRE and forms ternary complexes in the presence of *rev* and the RRE.[365] Two additional proteins have been recently isolated, apparently encoded on either human chromosome 6 or 12, of 120 and 62 kilodaltons.[366] Despite the description of these proteins, it still remained a question as to how *rev* rescues mRNA from the splicing process with the debate centering on nuclear export versus spliceosome disruption (or both). The description of B23's affinity for *rev* would hint that it participated in *rev*'s function by transportation of the *rev*:RRE complex out of the nucleus; and the descriptions of the other proteins were too preliminary to assign function. Additional data was accumulating, however, which pointed to disruption of spliceosome formation as the major mechanism protecting HIV-1 mRNA. This data was largely contributed by in vitro studies where nuclear export was not a factor. Kjems et al demonstrated a direct inhibition of splicing in vitro by *rev*; and moreover, showed that a 17 amino acid peptide corresponding to. the basic domain was also active in this inhibitory activity.[367] Extension of these early studies have demonstrated that *rev* blocks the assembly of U4,U5 and U6 small nuclear ribonucleoproteins (snRNPs) into the spliceosome apparatus.[368] Further, the more *rev* binding sites present within this assay system, the better the inhibition of assembly of these factors into spliceosomes, and the greater the inhibition to splicing.[368] It is interesting that this function maps to the basic domain (the RNA binding, nuclear localization, and multimerization region) rather than the activation domain which has been predicted to be the target for cellular protein interaction. One additional factor has been recently isolated which in fact does appear to interact with the activation domain and has been demonstrated to be the translation initiation factor 5A (eIF-5A).[369]

In summary, *rev* is an essential, virally determined, regulatory protein which results in the accumulation of singly spliced and unspliced HIV-1 mRNA species within the cytoplasm for translation. The protein has at least four functional domains: (i) the basic sequence specific-RNA binding region which physically overlaps the (ii) nuclear/ nucleolar localizing residues; and this basic region is flanked on both sides by the (iii) oligomerization domains (with some contribution from the activation domain) and (iv) the C-terminal activation domain characterized by a leucine-rich region that appears to be functionally interchangeable among many lentiviruses. This protein probably binds a single high affinity site defined by a 13 nucleotide "bubble" within the second stem loop of the RRE, whereupon, additional *rev* molecules accumulate on lower affinity sites and become stabilized either by *rev*:*rev* interaction or by *rev*:cellular protein interactions. This assembly of multiple *rev* molecules onto RRE-containing mRNAs either leads to: (i) efficient export from the nucleus prior to completion of splicing; or (ii) inhibition of the efficient assembly of certain components of the spliceosome; or (iii) through interaction with translational initiation factors and creation of stable association with polysomes; or

(iv) a combination of these events. The ultimate outcome is to shift the pattern of RNA expression from multiply-spliced, low molecular weight species to singly or unspliced, high molecular weight species.

While not specifically addressed in the above discussion, it is quite notable that this function of *rev* serves to down-regulate its own production by shifting from multiply-spliced mRNAs, from which *rev* is derived, to singly or unspliced species which exclude *rev*'s production. In fact, the temporal aspects of mRNA expression point to *rev* as the pivotal component to the pattern of protein expression[299,370] and therefore progeny virus production. *Rev* function has, in addition, been suggested to contribute to tissue specific levels of expression of virus resulting from its interaction with cell-specific proteins.[371] One could speculate teleologically, that this organization of the HIV-1 transcriptional repertoire offers the virus maximal advantage by allowing accumulation of the regulatory, non-surface expressed proteins early and thereby avoid flagging the cell for immune elimination. Once there is sufficient accumulation of these non-structural proteins, the *rev* "switch" can be thrown leading to rapid production of progeny virus. Once the *rev* "switch" is on, two outcomes can occur for the cell: either (i) immune destruction from HIV-1 specific cytotoxic T-cells or (ii) down-regulation of structural proteins as a result of loss of *rev* function with eclipsing of the infected cell from the immune system. This central role of *rev* in the viral life cycle makes it an ideal target for therapeutic intervention. One promising avenue of investigation has been the design and expression of intracellular single chain antibodies directed at the *rev* protein. Duan et al have shown dramatic reductions in virus production among many different acutely and chronically infected cell lines where this *rev*-specific antibody is expressed.[372] Whether the large reservoir of HIV-1 infected cells within patients can be targeted with this construct and therefore become of clinical utility remains an active area of research.

To briefly summarize the essential roles of these regulatory proteins in the determination of viral gene expression, *tat* functions to markedly increase the steady state level of viral transcripts and its level of expression in any given cell will dramatically affect the level of virus production within that cell. Much of *tat*'s function is attributed to its binding of the TAR region of RNA and promotion of efficient elongation of initiated transcripts,[204,374,375] however, it has also been reported to modestly increase the level of transcriptional initiation.[373] *Rev* is also an HIV-1 RNA binding protein which escorts these unspliced transcripts out of the nucleus where they can either be translated into polyproteins including the virion structural proteins or serve as genomic RNA for packaging.[233,367,377] In terms of latency these two regulatory proteins are critical to what we consider the second level of restriction (or latency) in HIV-1 infected cells which determines the fate of initiated viral transcripts. It has been established that a threshold level of *rev* is required to shift the pattern of RNA splicing to one in which the high molecular weight, genomic length species predominate;[299] and that the pattern of RNA splicing is distinctive to latently-infected cells where there is a predominance of the low molecular weight, multiply-spliced species as compared to productively-infected cells where there is a predominance of high molecular weight, unspliced viral RNA.[121,378-380] This pattern of RNA splicing has been correlated to primarily infected lymphocytes from patients at various stages of HIV-1 disease.[380] In some long term non-progressors, only very low levels of unspliced and multiply-spliced viral RNA species may be demonstrated in PBMCs.[376] In the early stages of disease there is usually a predominance of low molecular weight, multiply-spliced RNA consistent with the in vitro models;[121,378-380] (and S. Wolinsky personal communication with Pomerantz) and with progression of disease there is a shift to predominantly full length viral RNA.

LONG TERMINAL REPEAT (LTR)

The first level of restriction to viral gene expression is proviral transcriptional initiation. As with all retroviruses, HIV-1 has repeated sequences at both ends of its genome termed the long terminal repeat (LTR). The 5'LTR contains the majority of the DNA sequences required for the regulation of transcriptional activity of the virus; however, there is some evidence that there are intragenic enhancers that contribute modestly to the regulation of viral gene expression.[381-383] Figure 2.9 illustrates the organization of the 5' HIV-1 LTR with its regulatory elements. While somewhat arbitrary, the HIV-1 LTR can be divided into five functional regions: (i) the negative regulatory region; (ii) the enhancer or NF-κB sites; (iii) the Sp-1 sites; (iv) the TATA motif; and (v) the untranslated region including TAR.[384] The

Fig. 2.9. Simplified representation of the U3 and R region of the HIV-1 Long Terminal Repeat (LTR). The 5' region (i) of U3 contains multiple binding sites for cellular proteins and there is a tendency for deletions within this region to result in increased levels of viral gene expression. These observations are the origin of the designation of this region as the "negative regulatory element" or "modulatory region." The viral enhancer (ii) contains a perfect repeat of a decameric sequence which is established to bind the pleiotropic transcriptional factor nuclear factor-kappa B (NF-κB). The three Sp-1 sites (iii) and the TATA box with initiator element form the core (iv) promoter of HIV-1 and shares many similarities with "generic" cellular promoters. Immediately 3' to the transcriptional start site is the highly scrutinized TAR region, which upon transcription yields the highly structured RNA target for the tat protein.

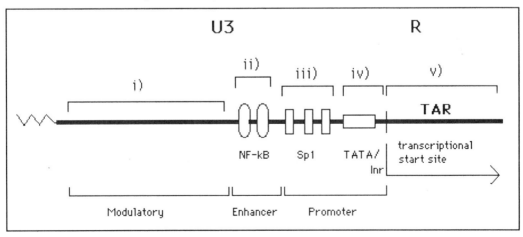

promoter (iii and iv above) of the HIV-1-LTR is similar to many cellular genes, in that it contains a TATA box immediately upstream of the transcriptional start site and a series of three short G + C rich regions which function as Sp-1 binding sites. An example of such similarity is the thyroid hormone response element.[385] Desai-Yajnik and Samuels established the presence of a thyroid response element within the NF-κB/Sp-1 region of the HIV-1 LTR which is transactivated by the thyroid hormone:receptor complex (T3R) to a similar magnitude as native thyroid hormone responsive genes.[385] In addition, in the presence of TAR, the T3R interaction with its cognate sequences become *tat* responsive; the efficient transactivation by T3R (in the absence of *tat*) is dependent upon both NF-κB sites; and as with the HIV-1 LTR discussed above (*tat* section), this *tat* responsiveness is Sp-1 site dependent.[273,385]

SP-1 BINDING SITES

The importance of the Sp-1 sites for basal and *tat*-induced LTR driven gene expression are well recognized.[229,386-391] Sequence analysis of the HIV-1 LTR shows three potential Sp-1 binding sites which have, in fact, been shown in vitro to bind purified Sp-1.[386,387] Mutational analysis of LTR constructs have demonstrated the requirement for at least one Sp-1 binding site for in vitro response to purified Sp-1.[386] Similarly, transient transfection of constructs containing mutations in these GC motifs demonstrate a gradient effect with loss of a small amount of basal and *tat*-induced activity in the presence of mutations in two of the three Sp-1 sites and essentially complete lack of activity with loss of all three sites.[387] Somewhat contradictory data was presented by Sakaguchi et al where in in vitro transcription reactions, they demonstrate that synthetic promoters consisting of either the TATA box alone or Sp-1 sites alone remain inducible with nuclear extracts from the PMA induced T-cell line CEM.[392] Similarly, a few reports of replication positive (albeit significantly less efficient) proviruses lacking all three Sp-1 sites have appeared;[388,389] however, these were deletions of Sp-1 sites and not mutations and it has been suggested that the NF-κB site, which has been moved significantly closer to the TATA box as a result of these deletions, may functionally substitute for Sp-1 binding in these mutant proviruses.[393] Perhaps the most relevant study of such mutants is that of Kim et al who created proviruses with linker substitutions within the LTR.[390] These constructs strictly maintain the spatial relationships throughout the LTR in contrast to deletional constructs. They showed essentially no viral replication in any of three cell lines tested with proviruses which lacked two of the three Sp-1 sites.[390] Similarly, site directed mutation of Sp-1 sites in proviral constructs has been reported to be non-replicative.[229] While the importance of Sp-1 binding sites to the efficient expression of HIV-1 gene products is well established, the precise mechanism of its transcriptional activation is poorly understood (in either LTR directed gene expression or cellular gene expression). The Sp-1 protein itself is a relatively large protein of 788 amino acids which contains three zinc finger motifs in its DNA binding region, multimerization sequences and an activation domain consisting of two glutamine-rich regions.[393-397] Upon binding, Sp-1 is phosphorylated by a DNA associated cellular kinase, the significance of which is unknown.[398] There is a suggestion that each GC box binds a tetramer of Sp-1 molecules and that with sequential Sp-1 binding sites as exist in the HIV-1 LTR there is further multimerization of these tetramers to form large complexes.[395,396] It is further suggested that this large protein:DNA complex results in DNA looping;[396,399] and that this looping approximates transcriptional factors located long distances upstream with the basic promoter element, resulting in transcriptional activation. Alternatively, for HIV-1, there is evidence that the cooperative interaction between the upstream enhancer, NF-κB, and Sp-1 results from direct protein:protein interaction between adjacent binding sites.[400] Perkins et al show that mutation of neighboring NF-κB and Sp-1 sites abrogate the synergistic effects of these two functional units; that their physical interaction as demonstrated by electrophoretic mobility shift assays is cooperative; and that the exact spatial and orientational parameters must be maintained for their functional interaction.[400]

Traditional discussions of control mechanisms of gene expression include a consideration of the promoter's methylation state.[401,402] Since methylation occurs preferentially at GC islands, Sp-1 binding sites are potential targets for methylation. Preliminary data from several laboratories have suggested that DNA methylation of the HIV-1 promoter plays some role in restricting viral gene expression.[403-405] 5-azacytidine, a DNA methyltransferase inhibitor has been shown to increase the level of LTR-driven gene expression in stable integrated plasmid constructs; and conversely, in vitro methylation of the HIV-1 promoter has been shown to decrease expression.[403-405] Two potential mechanisms have been suggested to mediate this repression of gene expression. One mechanism may be the masking of DNA binding sites by the protruding methyl group resulting in an inefficient protein:DNA interaction; and an alternative mechanism is the preferential binding of a cellular repressive factor(s) recognizing the altered GC site(s).[406-409] A recent study by Joel et al has demonstrated such a potentially repressive factor for HIV-1 methylated Sp-1 sites.[410] They describe this protein, HIV-1 methylated DNA binding protein (HMBP), to bind as a dimer at Sp-1 sites of the HIV-1 LTR preferentially when the Sp-1 sites are methylated; and demonstrate its presence in nuclear extracts from human T cells and HeLa cells.[410] Functional analysis of this new protein remains to be reported. It should also be mentioned that methylation of GC dinucleotides at sites other than Sp-1 sites in the HIV-1 LTR may contribute to reduced viral gene expression.[411] Bednarik et al have shown interference with binding of NF-κB to its cognate sites if the GC dinucleotide positioned between the two NF-κB sites is methylated.[411]

In addition to the Sp-1 protein, an additional cellular factor has been recently described which binds GC boxes including those of the HIV-1 LTR.[397,412] This factor, termed BTEB, is substantially smaller than Sp-1; however, not surprisingly, this protein shares significant sequence homology with the DNA binding portion of Sp-1 and is expressed in many tissues including lymphoid tissue.[397] Transient transfection of a BTEB expressing plasmid into cells containing an LTR driven reporter gene resulted in increased transcriptional activity both in the presence and absence of *tat* and was shown to act cooperatively with NF-κB sites, as does Sp-1.[400,412] Because essentially all cells express Sp-1, it is difficult to examine the effects of BTEB in isolation outside of in vitro transcription assays utilizing purified transcriptional factors. It is difficult to imagine how this molecule participates in the complex assembly of the transcriptional machinery onto the HIV-1 promoter. Studies to determine the relative abundance of Sp-1 and BTEB molecules bound to these GC motifs under various states of transcriptional activity will be important to dissect each protein's contribution. It could be speculated that given the substantially smaller size of BTEB, it has fewer potential surfaces to contact other proteins and might therefore be less efficient at stabilizing proteins bound to flanking sequences as proposed for Sp-1;[393] or to be less efficient at multimerization as demonstrated for Sp-1.[395,396,399]

THE TATA BOX AND INITIATOR ELEMENTS

A great deal has been learned about the generic TATA box which is widely utilized by viral and cellular genes. These elements, generally positioned about 30 base pairs upstream of the transcriptional start site, appear to function as the "staging area" for most RNA polymerase II directed transcription. The TATA sequence serves as the nidus for assembly of an ever growing number of transcriptional factors (and co-factors) which comprise the pre-initiation complex.[413-417] The TATA sequence itself is recognized and bound by the TATA binding protein (TBP) which is a component of the transcription factor TFIID; this is followed by the recruitment of the transcription factors TFIIA, TFIIB, TFIIE, TFIIF, TFIIH, TFIIG/TFII-IJ[415,418-421] and some recently described co-factors.[422,423] Mutational analysis of the HIV-1 LTR TATA and flanking sequences demonstrate their importance in regulation of HIV-1 gene expression.[176,212,424] Despite their generic appearance and function, it is becoming clear that not all TATA boxes are equivalent. It has been shown that substituting the TATA element from SV40 or other cellular promoters markedly reduces transcriptional initiation from the HIV-1 LTR.[229] Since it would appear that the same general group of transcriptional factors (the TFII-series) are utilized by all of these TATA elements, it is not entirely clear why there should be such a requirement for its own TATA element for efficient usage by the HIV-1 LTR. In addition to affecting the basal level of transcriptional initiation from the LTR, the HIV-1 TATA box is necessary to maintain *tat* responsiveness.[211] As discussed above (*tat* section) this TATA element is necessary for formation of the non-processive transcriptional complexes which are, in fact, the complexes that are *tat* responsive.[211] One possible explanation for such an effect is the identification of a poorly characterized upstream stimulatory activity (USA) which is present within this region of the HIV-1 LTR.[425] This factor leads to increased transcriptional activity presumably by improving the protein:protein interactions between the general transcriptional factors assembled onto the

TATA sequence and the Sp-1 proteins assembled onto their cognate sequences immediately upstream.[393,425] It is becoming clear that transcriptional initiation from the HIV-1 LTR (as well as cellular promoters) involves the recruitment of an enormous complex of DNA-bound proteins which interact with each other over a long distance. One model to accommodate all of the above data is shown in Figure 2.10. The 12 Sp-1 molecules are bridged by an HIV-1 LTR specific factor, USA, to the large pre-initiation complex which occurs over the span of ap-

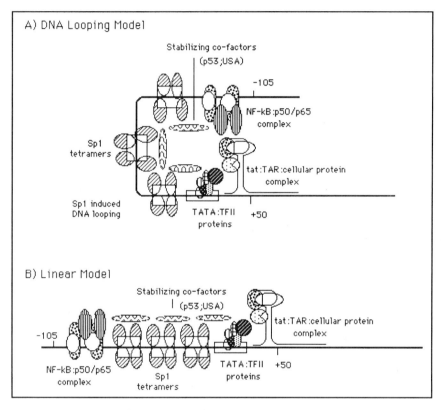

Fig. 2.10. Two models of the assembly of the pre-initiation complex. One of the emerging themes in transcriptional regulation is the concept of stability of the protein:protein:DNA interactions that take place immediately upstream of the transcriptional start site. Certainly one aspect of this stability is contributed by the tertiary structure of these complexes. Sp-1 binding has been associated with DNA looping which may provide one mechanism to bring upstream enhancer binding proteins into close proximity with other critical elements of the transcriptional machinery. In panel A, this DNA looping is hypothesized to bring the NF-κB complex in close proximity with not only the TATA binding transcriptional factors but with the assembled tat:TAR:cellular protein complex. These associations might, in turn, be stabilized by the presence of other factors such as USA or wild type p53. It might be further hypothesized that this highly structured protein:DNA complex leads to the formation of the "processive" transcripts depicted in Figure 2.5C. By comparison, in panel B, we might speculate that an "assembly line" effect is present in which each adjacent protein:DNA contact results in the stabilization of its neighboring protein:DNA contact, ultimately resulting in a downstream stabilization of "generic" transcriptional factors leading to transcriptional processivity. There is insufficient data to support one of these hypotheses over the other at the present time; and indeed, a totally different mechanism may be involved in the cellular "decision" to form one complex over the other.

proximately 60-70 base pairs (and including the initiator complex—
see below). In addition, the *tat*:TAR:cellular protein complex as discussed above is now brought into proximity to this complex where
there is probably some physical interaction between either *tat* itself
(i.e. with TFIIF) or a cellular protein assembled with *tat* and this large
protein: DNA complex. This interaction might be predicted to change
the architecture of some part or even the whole of the Sp-1/TATA
structure resulting in the establishment of a processive transcriptional
complex rather a non-processive complex (see *tat* section above).

To complicate this picture further is the recent data on the effect
of the proto-oncogene p53 on HIV-1 gene expression from this minimal Sp-1/TATA promoter.[426,427] Duan et al and Subler et al independently demonstrated that mutant p53 (as occurs in a number of ma-
lignancies) increases transcription from the HIV-1 LTR and that wild
type p53 inhibits transcriptional activity. This effect was particularly
marked in the presence of the minimal promoter of Sp-1/TATA. When
NF-κB sites were included, the inhibitory effect of wild type p53 and
the stimulatory effect of mutant p53 were diminished as they were in
the presence of *tat*:TAR.[426,427] Furthermore, introduction of a retroviral
vector expressing mutant p53 into U1 cells which completely lack
endogenous p53 resulted in up-regulation of viral replication. In contrast, introduction of this vector into the cell line ACH-2 which *does*
express endogenous mutant p53 had no effect.[426] The model proposed
for these observations is the stabilization of protein:protein interactions among the assembled group of proteins on this stretch of DNA
encompassing the Sp-1 sites and the TATA element.[426,427] Under basal
levels of transcriptional activity (in the absence of transactivation by
either NF-κB or *tat*) wild type p53 might be expected to help maintain restricted viral gene expression. In the presence of a mutant p53,
this repressive activity is lost and even perhaps replaced by a stimulatory effect. It is interesting to speculate that one reason for the high
level of expression of HIV-1 viral mRNA in the adenocarcinoma biopsy discussed above is the loss of wild type p53 (see page 16). It is
also once again pointed out that there are multiple contributions to
HIV-1 latency in that U1 cells and ACH-2 cells responded differently
to expression of mutant p53.[426]

Further insight into the importance of this regulatory element in
HIV-1 is gained from an analysis of second site revertants. Ross et al
reported viral growth patterns of selected mutant viruses lacking Sp-1
sites and demonstrated a wide range of permissiveness depending upon
the cell type being infected.[389] Parenthetically, this spectrum of replicative potential probably results from the complex assembly of the many
cellular factors as outlined above, with some cells better than others at
compensating the loss of Sp-1 sites in their assembly of competent
pre-initiation complexes. Of further interest was the late outgrowth of
some viruses even from the non-permissive cells.[428] Sequence analysis
of these phenotypic revertants revealed that while they maintained their
original Sp-1 mutations, they had gained mutations immediately upstream of the TATA box. These new "improved" TATA elements had
no effect when placed in the context of wild type HIV-1 LTRs, how-

ever, they restored function to mutant LTRs lacking functional Sp-1 sites. They further characterized these revertant sequences and showed that they resulted in an increased stability of the general transcription factors TFIIA and TFIID assembled onto their target DNA.[428]

In addition to the TATA box, many cellular and viral promoters have a poorly defined functional region immediately downstream which is termed the initiator element (Inr).[424,429-431] This was originally described for a TATA-less promoter but has subsequently been identified in a number of TATA containing promoters, including that of HIV-1.[424,431] HIV-1 has been reported to contain two such elements, one from position -2 to +8 and another from +32 to +41. Mutations within the putative HIV-1 initiator sequences from -2 to +8 have been demonstrated to down-regulate HIV-1 expression.[434] Two cellular proteins have been described which interact with other cellular initiators and may participate in regulation of HIV-1 through its Inr sequence. One is a member of the TFII-family of proteins termed TFII-I; and appears to be closely related to the USF factor which binds an upstream motif in HIV-1 (discussed below).[431] The other protein is the YY1 protein. Initially described as a transcriptional repressor in an adeno-associated virus, several subsequent reports describe YY1 as a transcriptional activator.[429,432,433] In the setting of the HIV-1 LTR, YY1 appears to behave similarly to that of the adeno-associated viral system, in that overexpression of the protein results in down-regulation of LTR directed gene expression.[434]

The basic core promoter of HIV-1, then, consists of the three Sp-1 sites followed closely by the TATA element with an associated initiator sequence. It is this region of the HIV-1 promoter which determines the basal level of transcription. Despite some differences between different TATA boxes, it is apparent that control of basal levels of transcription from the integrated HIV-1 provirus is not dramatically different from control of many other cellular genes. It is also likely, that the ultimate transcriptional activity of this or any other promoter is the consequence of the stability of these assembled protein:DNA complexes; and that this stability is determined by the relative contribution of each of the many different factors (and co-factors) involved. From this scenario then, it could be imagined that there is a spectrum of basal HIV-1 transcription within any given cell which is determined by both the level (and perhaps even the kind) of endogenous general transcriptional factors such as the TFII-series of protein, the Sp-1 multimers and initiator proteins. These levels of endogenous transcriptional factors may in turn be influenced by the metabolic state of the infected cell (i.e. activated T cells versus quiescent T cells). In addition, the relative access of these factors to their cognate sequences as determined by integration site and chromatin organization (see below and chapter 3) may add to this spectrum of activity.

NUCLEAR FACTOR-KAPPA B (NF-κB) AND THE HIV-1 ENHANCER

Beyond the above core promoter of HIV-1, as with many other regulated cellular genes, the HIV-1 LTR contains an enhancer element. Upstream of the Sp-1 sites are the duplicated NF-κB binding sites, defined by the sequence GGGACTTTCC, which have commanded a great deal of attention in that they strongly regulate transcriptional initiation from the HIV-1-LTR.[393,435-437] Initially described as a B-cell specific transcriptional factor,[438] NF-κB is now recognized as a member of the *rel* family of transcriptional factors and is found in nearly all eukaryotic cells where it is complexed in the cytoplasm with its inhibitor, I-κB, in an inactive form (see below).[439-441] Since NF-κB's initial recognition as a potent *trans*-activator of HIV-1 gene expression, there have been tremendous strides made in unraveling the molecular biology of this/these factor(s) (reviewed in ref. 442). The prototypic NF-κB factor is a heterodimer of a p50 and p65 subunit.[443,445] The p50 subunit is derived from a precursor protein of 105 kilodaltons which is processed by cellular enzymes and, interestingly, has been shown to be a substrate for HIV-1's protease.[446-449] This 50 kilodalton protein is capable of forming homodimers in addition to heterodimers with p65 and these homodimers can bind and in some contexts, activate transcription from NF-κB binding sequences.[450-452] Of note, the prototypic I-κB binding site for the heterodimer lies within the p65 subunit and therefore I-κB is ineffective at sequestering p50 homodimers.[450,451,453] The p65 subunit of this transcriptional factor has also been shown to form homodimers which can bind these specific sites (albeit with lower affinity) and result in transcriptional activation.[450] Both of these proteins contain regions of high homology to the v-rel viral oncogene and its cellular homologue c-rel; and all of this family of proteins including p50 and p65 can presumably complex in various combinations with each other through these regions of homology which also define the DNA binding domain.[452-455] While the prototypic NF-κB transcriptional factor is a potent transactivator of HIV-1, it is unclear what role the various combinations of proteins play in determining the level of HIV-1 gene expression. It has been determined that these different protein complexes have differing affinities for their target NF-κB sites.[456] In vitro transcriptional systems, which allow better control of these protein:protein associations, have provided some additional insight into NF-κB's mechanism of transactivation.[450,457] One interesting finding has been the recent demonstration of NF-κB's dependence upon the newly described USA co-factor for its transactivation potential in vitro.[457] In addition, while earlier data suggested that both homodimers of p50 and p65 could bind and transactivate transcription, in vitro studies with purified subunits show their mechanisms of action to be distinct. It would appear that the p50 homodimer is very effective at DNA binding but must assume a certain three-dimensional configuration for successful transactivation.[450] In contrast, homodimers of p65 are less effective at target binding and have a transactivation domain (residing in its carboxy terminal region) distinct from the v-rel homologous sequences.[450] The establishment of an active p50 homodimer is determined by the precise sequence to which it is bound, being most active when bound to the NF-κB sites of the class I major histocompatability complex genes. It has been suggested that while p50 homodimers (originally isolated as the MHC class I transcriptional factor

KBF-1) recognizes nearly all NF-κB sites, only within the precise sequence context of MHC-class I does it assume the chymotrypsin resistant conformation that exposes its activating domain(s).[442,450,452] In contrast, p65 homodimer transactivation is not dependent upon DNA induced protein conformation but is dependent upon DNA binding affinity; that is, the higher the binding affinity of p65 to its target the greater the transactivating potential.[450] In the context of heterodimerization of p50 and p65, it appears that each moiety contributes independently to its effects (although p65's contribution is probably greater).[442,450,458] Furthermore, the DNA binding affinity of the heterodimer is intermediate to that of the respective homodimers with the p50 homodimer having the highest affinity and p65 the lowest; however, in the presence of equimolar ratios of p50 and p65, there is evidence of a strong preference for heterodimer formation rather than homodimer formation.[450,457] It would be predicted from these observations, and has been suggested, that in cellular environments in which there is molar excess of p50, there is homodimerization which results in its binding to the HIV-1 LTR but without activation because of a lack of the required conformational change.[459-461] This could conceivably result in an inhibitory effect if its binding now precludes binding of the p50/p65 heterodimer. In U1 cells which have been used as a model of latency (determined by cellular millieu rather than integration site), there is evidence for a predominance of p50 homodimer formation in the unstimulated state.[130] Upon stimulation, which results in markedly increased viral gene expression, there is a shift to what appears to be the prototypic p50/p65 heterodimer.[130] In further support of such a competitive nature of these related proteins is the demonstration by Doerre et al that overexpression of c-rel in the nucleus blocks the up-regulation of HIV-1 expression upon induction of free NF-κB.[462] Furthermore, this inhibitory effect is dependent upon the DNA binding (rel homology region) domain of c-rel, suggesting that c-rel is competing with NF-κB for occupancy of the NF-κB sites.[462] Bcl-3 is another rel-related protein which has been demonstrated to preferentially bind and remove inhibitory p50 homodimers from their target thereby allowing access of p50/p65 heterodimers to their target with subsequent transactivation.[459]

Finally, another related protein (termed either p49 or p52) is derived from a precursor p100 protein and appears to function similarly to p50, in that it can bind p65 and transactivate NF-κB sites; has significant rel homology; and is formed by the proteolytic cleavage of its precursor.[446,463-465] The precise role that this protein plays in NF-κB transactivation is still evolving. Deciphering the precise role of each of these many potential protein:protein and protein:DNA interactions in the overall level of expression of HIV-1 and their contribution in vivo to cellular latency remain to be determined; however, the relative contribution of each will likely depend upon the specific cellular system under investigation.

While the remarkable complexity of this pleiotropic transcriptional factor lends itself to an equally complex role in the regulation of many cellular genes, a great deal of evidence supports its role as a significant transactivator of HIV-1 gene expression. Adding an additional incre-ment of complexity to its function, is the interaction of NF-κB with its inhibitor I-κB. There have been two proteins cloned which possess prototypic I-κB activity: MAD-3 and pp40.[465,467] MAD-3 is the prod-uct of a rapidly induced mRNA initially isolated from macrophages in response to adherence.[465,467] MAD-3 and pp40 both have five repeats of an ankyrin related sequence; and of particular interest is the find-ing that the carboxy terminal region (CTR) of the p50 subunit pre-cursor, p105, has seven of these ankyrin like repeats; and in fact inde-pendent expression of this CTR portion of the p105 molecule produces a protein with I-κB-like activity.[465-467] Furthermore, for functional ex-pression of p50, this CTR needs to be removed by cellular (or viral) proteases.[447] This has lead to the speculation that one mechanism of control of p50 function is at the level of this proteolytic step and as mentioned above, acute infection with HIV-1 can lead to an increase in this proteolytic process.[447] Whether the liberation of this moiety creates the I-κB responsible for sequestration of p50/p65 in the cyto-plasm remains an open question; however, at least one study demon-strates the rapid destruction of the newly liberated CTR after its pro-teolytic removal. In addition, the CTR moiety of p105 has a higher affinity for the p50 subunit than for the p65 subunit of NF-κB which is unlike the prototypic I-κB molecule; and independent in vitro ex-pression of CTR creates a protein capable of binding and sequester-ing, in *trans*, p50 in the cytoplasm.[468,469] On the other hand, circum-stantial evidence of the functional similarity of this CTR with I-κB is the recent demonstration of the rapid destruction of the I-κB protein after its phosphorylation in response to stimuli which liberate NF-κB.[470] It may be that the CTR is functioning in *cis* and in *trans* with p50 while it (or more likely a similar protein such as I-κB/MAD-3) is func-tioning in *trans* with p65; and that free CTR and I-κB are inherently unstable when not in the presence of NF-κB accounting for their rapid destruction. Finally, NF-κB has been shown to up-regulate the pro-duction of its own p50 subunit precursor, p105.[471] This could offer a feedback mechanism for overexpression of p50 leading to homo-dimerization and transdominant inhibition of NF-κB sites to "shut down" the genes previously activated by NF-κB. On the other hand, it might replace the pool of intact p105 molecules which are awaiting rapid induction through the proteolytic cleavage process.

In summary then, the inhibitors of NF-κB are beginning to take on the same complexity as their target NF-κB molecules. At present, it appears that the CTR and Bcl-3 members of this family have a greater affinity for the p50 subunit of NF-κB while the pp40, I-κB-α (MAD-3) and I-κB-β have greater affinity for the p65 subunit. What these molecules all share however, is the high number of repeated ankyrin sequences. Whether these ankyrin motifs function in these molecules as they are proposed to in ankyrin (that is, binding cytoskeletal ele-ments) remains to be determined. Regardless of the precise mecha-nism, these elements all interact with their targets to inactivate their respective transcriptional activity, illustrating again the incremental nature of the transcriptional process with its multiple "checks and balances."

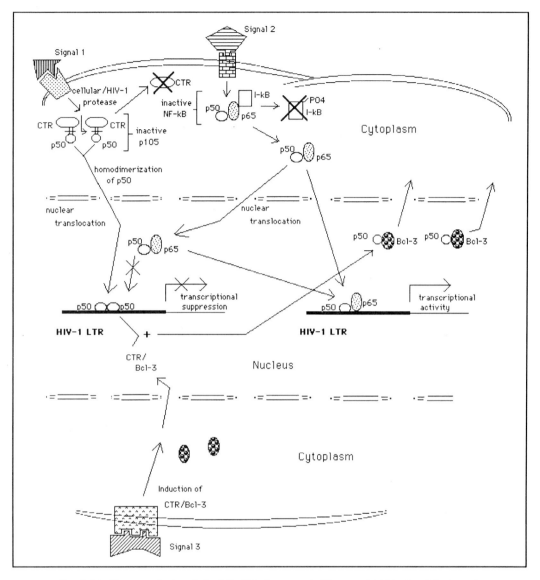

Fig. 2.11. The complexity of the NF-κB/I-κB system is illustrated. With signal 1, there is activation of the proteolytic process which releases the p50 subunit of NF-κB from its cis acting CTR, creating a molar excess of p50. This molar excess of p50 leads to homodimerization and nuclear translocation (without its cytoplasmic targeting domain, CTR). The p50 homodimer recognizes the decameric NF-κB target sequence where it binds but fails to transactivate the downstream gene unless it assumes the chymotrypsin resistant configuration (determined by the context of the bound DNA). Signal 2 leads to activation of a cellular kinase system with phosporylation of I-κB leading to dissociation from the prototypic p50/p65 heterodimer and rapid destruction of I-κB. The p50/p65 heterodimer is translocated to the nucleus where, in the absence of a binding site competitor such as p50/p50, it binds its target and leads to gene expression. In the presence of p50 homodimers, p50/p65 is ineffective at binding its target with resultant restriction of gene expression. With signal 3, there is induction of excess CTR or Bcl-3 and removal of p50 homodimers. In the presence of signal 2 and signal 3, the p50/p65 heterodimers is again able to engage its target with transcriptional activation. All of the above is of course tempered by the vast number of other protein:DNA interactions which are occurring outside of this core enhancer region.

There are multiple environmental stimuli which lead to the liberation of NF-κB from its inhibitor, including lipopolysaccharide (LPS),[472] PMA,[473,474] PHA,[475] H_2O_2,[476,477] tumor necrosis factor-alpha (TNF-α),[125,478] leukemia inhibitory factor,[479] alkylating agents,[490] phosphatidylcholine hydrolysis,[481] and certain viral infections,[482-484] all of which have been shown to increase LTR-directed gene expression, primarily in transient transfection assays and transformed cell lines. While not absolutely essential to viral replication,[392,485,486] loss of this repeated 10 bp sequence markedly reduces viral gene expression in most cells.[487-490] Although initially described as the target of a tissue-specific transcriptional factor, it has become clear over the last few years that the NF-κB binding motif is found in multiple cellular genes and is recognized by proteins and protein complexes other than the prototypic p50/p65 form of this transcriptional factor.[444,491-495] In addition to binding NF-κB, these 10 bp repeats have been described to bind: HIVEN 86A (in activated T-cells and which has been subsequently shown to be identical to c-rel);[448,496] EBP-1 in quiescent T-cells;[497] H2TF1 in the regulation of class I major histocompatibility complex genes;[498] and TCIIB in SV40 infected cells.[499] Two additional factors, ETS and MBP-1/PRDII-BF1, have been more extensively studied and may have a potential impact on HIV-1 expression.

MBP-1/PRDII-BF1 belongs to a large family of DNA binding proteins containing zinc-finger binding motifs.[501,502] MBP-1/PRDII-BF1 is a 300 kilodalton protein which contains two NF-κB binding domains which are widely spaced.[501,502] Each of these two binding domains can be expressed independently by alternative splicing to yield proteins of 200 and 68 kilodaltons, both of which retain their DNA binding ability.[502] In addition to binding the NF-κB sequences, the full length protein also binds TAR region DNA in the loop defining region.[503] While the significance of this remains undefined, one speculation is that this protein might serve to approximate the DNA between the two binding sites; although it is difficult to imagine how approximating the DNA between TAR and NF-κB would benefit viral gene expression. In addition to demonstrating that MBP-1/PRDII-BF1 can bind the NF-κB motif from the HIV-1 LTR, Seeler et al also demonstrated that it can stimulate LTR directed gene expression; and suggested that the smaller, single site proteins might act to competitively inhibit NF-κB's transactivation of the LTR.[503]

The second family of transcriptional factors with binding specificities within the HIV-1 LTR NF-κB motifs is the ETS family of proteins.[504,505] There are several proteins within this family including ETS1, ETS2, ERG, ERGB/Hu-FLI-1 and ELF1. Most of these proteins are expressed within cells of hematopoetic origin.[504] ETS1 and ETS2 have been shown to bind and transactivate the HTLV-I and MSV retroviral LTRs.[506,507] This family of transcriptional factors is more traditional in that they contain a single DNA binding domain and a single transactivating domain.[504] Unlike MBP-1/PRDII-BF1, which recognizes the decameric NF-κB sequence, the minimal binding site for ETS proteins is contained within the four nucleotide GGAA sequence in the 3' end of the decameric sequence (in the antisense orientation).

Seth et al demonstrated that members of this ETS family of proteins not only bind but also transactivate the HIV-1 LTR.[508] Furthermore, they found that a single nucleotide substitution flanking this minimal site in the Z2Z6 viral isolate conferred a 40-fold increase in transactivating potential compared with HXB2.[508] It is tempting to speculate that since such a minimal change (a single nucleotide) can so markedly change transcriptional activity in response to this protein, that such minor changes within key regions belie the different replicative phenotypes of different viruses.

In summary then, the core enhancer of the HIV-1 LTR has been established beyond a reasonable doubt to be a critical participant in determining the level of transcriptional activity from the integrated provirus. As more is learned about the molecular biology of NF-κB and other transcriptional factors recognizing the decameric NF-κB consensus sequences, it is clear that they paint a remarkably complex picture of transcriptional regulation. While the depth of understanding of the participants involved in this process is gratifying, it is daunting to construct all of the possible scenarios of assembly of the many potential protein:protein and protein:DNA interactions; and even more daunting to then make predictions of their effect on transcriptional activity. Add to this complexity, the subtleties of assembly of transcriptional factors and co-factors associated with the Sp-1 sites, TATA box and initiator element and it is no wonder that the "magic bullet" to specifically interrupt HIV-1 transcription without disrupting the regulation of critical cellular genes has yet to be discovered.

THE NEGATIVE REGULATORY ELEMENT

Upstream of the NF-κB binding sequences is a less precisely defined region termed the negative regulatory element (NRE) of the LTR reviewed in.[158,383,509] It has been shown in vitro and in vivo that deletion of this region of the LTR results in an increase in the level of viral gene expression (albeit a modest increase).[487-489,510] Within this region of the LTR are a number of sites recognized by cellular factors. As depicted in Figure 2.12, there are two AP-1[511] binding sites in addition to a binding site for nuclear factor of activated T-cells (NFAT-1) within this region.[512,513] Deletion of these AP-1 binding sites by themselves, however, has little effect on viral gene expression.[510] By contrast, the binding sequences for USF (upstream binding factor) and NFAT-1 appear to down-regulate viral gene expression in that their deletion leads to increased viral replication as well as LTR driven reporter gene expression.[510,514] Upstream binding factor (USF) is a 43-50 kilodalton protein which contains features of the helix-loop-helix family of transcriptional proteins; it recognizes a minimal DNA sequence of CACGTG; and it has been shown to bind to the HIV-1 LTR.[515-517] In addition to USF, other helix-loop-helix transcriptional factors recognize this specific sequence and may therefore participate in HIV-1's transcriptional regulation. Of particular interest are the Myc and Max proteins.[518] These proteins work cooperatively to "fine tune" expression from this CACGTG enhancer motif when placed upstream of a core promoter (as it occurs in HIV-1).[518] Max is capable of homodimerization as well as heterodimerization with Myc. When Myc is overexpressed, there is transcriptional up-regulation which is dependent upon its binding to this sequence. When Max is overexpressed, there is repression of transcription, also dependent upon its DNA binding site. One can overcome this transcriptional repression by overexpression of Myc which in turn is dependent upon its dimerization site.[518] These observations would suggest that this tandem protein interaction can either stimulate or repress transcription depending upon their molar ratios, reminiscent of the p50:p65 relationship of NF-κB. While it is not determined that Myc:Max participate in the regulation of HIV-1 gene expression, the potential exists for yet another intricate protein: protein:DNA interaction to contribute to this regulation.

While relatively little is known of USF's specific effect on HIV-1 LTR, its function in other transcriptional units suggest a novel activity. There is mounting evidence that chromatin structural organization plays a significant role in the transcriptional control of many genes (discussed in detail in chapter 3). This might be expected to be particularly relevant with HIV-1 whose proviral sequences are maintained within the context of the host cell's chromatin structure. In the setting of in vitro chromatin assembly, USF has been shown to act in concert with TFIID in the competition between assembly of promoters into transcriptionally silent nucleosomes versus assembly into transcriptionally competent pre-initiation complexes.[519] This effect is present only if USF is present prior to nucleosome assembly and in the presence of TFIID. The presence of USF during chromatin assembly results in a greater number of promoters which contain transcriptionally competent pre-initiation complexes; however, once these pre-initiation complexes are formed in the presence of USF, the percentage that went on to transcriptional activity was independent of USF.[519] It would appear from these observations that USF might function by preventing the down-regulation of LTR function that would result from the assembly of this DNA into transcriptionally silent nucleosome structures. There is at least preliminary evidence that in fact this region of the LTR is maintained in a nucleosome free configuration. Verdin mapped DNase I hypersensitivity sites along the HIV-1 LTR in several chronically infected cell lines.[383] He reported a nucleosome free region extending from around the transcriptional start site through (and past) the USF site.[383] Of note, even in the uninduced state where there was little transcriptional activity, the core enhancer and basic promoter region remained protected from nucleolytic cleavage.[383] This would suggest that the NF-κB sites and possible Sp-1/TATA sites were occupied.

These observations were independently corroborated by ligation mediated PCR analysis of methylation protection patterns in U1 cells.[520] Very interestingly, in addition to the core enhancer remaining protected from methylation, (suggesting pre-bound transcriptional factors as above) the USF sequences were specifically covered, presumably by USF, and this protection was independent of transcriptional stimulation.[520] While too early to conclude that the USF transcriptional factor is functioning in the HIV-1 LTR (perhaps in conjunction with TBP/TFIID) by preventing the incorporation of these sequences into transcriptionally repressed chromatin structures, this data is compatible with such a function. Another element recently identified in the GAL4 transcriptional system of yeast is the nucleosomal displacement sequence ACCCG.[521,522] As more fully discussed in chapter 3, this short sequence was shown to result in an approximately 230 base pair stretch of DNA lacking in nucleosome condensation regardless of the context into which it was placed.[521,522] Of particular interest in this regard is the presence of this sequence immediately upstream of the NF-AT binding site in the HIV-1 LTR (unpublished observation-ML).

Zeichner et al constructed a series of linker scanner mutants extending through most of the U3 region of the HIV-1 LTR.[490] They substituted an 18 base pair sequence for the wild type sequence sequentially from position -453 through +15. With each 18 base pair substitution, they maintained the wild type sequence in the remainder of the LTR. Through a series of transient transfection studies they then analyzed the effect on transcription of each 18 base pair region of the LTR.[490,523,524] With the exception of the core enhancer and basic promoter region, the effects observed further upstream were quite variable depending upon the cell system into which these constructs were transfected and also of relatively small magnitude.[250,523,524] In an attempt to further evaluate those mutants covering the negative regulatory element in the context of a natural infection, Kim et al placed a selected few of these mutant LTRs into a background of the viral isolate pNL4-3.[390] Interestingly, in peripheral blood lymphocytes and in the cell line 11.8, all but one of these mutant LTRs severely damaged the replicative capacity of the new virus. Only the mutant with the altered LTR from position -166 to -183 had replication kinetics similar to the wild type virus.[390] This region encompasses the upstream most portion of the USF region (although five of the six core recognition nucleotides CACGTG for USF binding were maintained). By contrast, the mutant -148 to -165 which eliminates five of these six nucleotides was severely damaged (as were other mutants not encompassing the USF region).[609] It is difficult to provide a precise mechanism for these findings where it would appear that the negative regulatory region is in fact acting as a positive regulatory element. One conclusion to be drawn, however, is that interpretation of transient transfection assays need to be tempered in the context of natural infection with HIV-1.

Another recently described transcriptional factor which appears in vitro to transactivate the HIV-1 LTR from the *negative* regulatory element is NF-IL6. Tesmer et al demonstrated several potential binding sites for NF-IL6 within the HIV-1 LTR, one of which partially overlaps the minimal sequence for USF binding; unfortunately, it also binds to two other sites with somewhat discordant sequences.[525] Furthermore, NF-IL6 has been recently demonstrated to bind the p50 subunit of NF-κB independent of prior DNA binding by either factor.[526] It is interesting that one of the second sites which appeared to bind NF-IL6 is in fact immediately adjacent to an NF-κB site which might function as adjoining target sites for a p50:NF-IL6 heterodimer with increased stability. Finally, there also appears to be a physical interaction between NF-IL6 and the p65 subunit of NF-κB in the transactivation of the IL6 gene.[527]

Less well characterized factor binding sites include a 10 bp sequence (-175 through -185) that resembles a repressor sequence in yeast termed upstream repressor sequence (URS);[528] and site B which is a palindromic sequence that binds a 100 kilodalton protein abundant in T-lymphocytes. This factor (COUP-TF) has been shown to down-regulate viral transcription and is related to the family of binding sites for steroid/thyroid hormone receptor complexes.[529-531] A short distance upstream of the NF-κB sites within the negative regulatory regions is a binding sequence for TCF1α. This T-cell specific transcriptional factor contains a 68 amino acid region with high homology to the high mobility group (HMG) proteins which are non-histone, DNA binding proteins.[532-534] It is interesting that the high mobility group protein HMG I(Y) has been shown to be essential to the NF-κB mediated up-regulation of the human interferon-β (IFN-β) gene in response to viral infection.[535] It might be that TCF1α's close proximity to the NF-κB sites within the HIV-1 LTR allow it to function similarly to HMG I(Y) in the IFN-β enhancer. While no direct effect on HIV-1 gene expression has yet been demonstrated for TCF1α, comparison of primary isolates with a spontaneous duplication of the TCF1α binding region showed increased replication kinetics in T lymphocytes.[536]

While it is clear that the promoter/enhancer regions, (NF-κB sites, Sp-1 binding sites, the TATA sequence, and initiator element), are clearly involved in transcriptional regulation, the overall significance of this "negative regulatory element" (with its multiple potential binding sites) to HIV-1 viral gene expression remains to be defined. Much of the data accumulated to date is contradictory, is of small magnitude, or is restricted to a defined cellular system. Given these findings it is tempting to dismiss the importance of this region of the HIV-1 LTR; however, past experience would caution against doing so. It was difficult to attribute much, if any, function to the *nef* genes of SIV/ HIV after extensive study in vitro. Its importance was only appreciated following the demonstration of its requirement for disease progression in the SIV animal model.[537,538] Sequence data from primary isolates of HIV-1 suggest significant conservation within this region and it is therefore very likely to serve some essential function in vivo; and since there are no protein products derived from this region (at least in the 5'LTR) we are left to assume it functions in some transcriptional regulatory capacity. One intriguing recent report, however, does demonstrate a higher mutation rate in the U3 region of the SIV LTR in the absence of a functionally expressed *nef* gene (i.e. containing a deletion within the region upstream of the 3'LTR).[539] Whether the negative regulatory element of the U3 region of the 5'LTR is maintained as an "artifact" of the retroviral replication mechanism (i.e. duplication of the 3'LTR) and merely reflects its use in the 3'LTR to generate *nef* proteins remains to be determined.

THE TAR ELEMENT DNA

Downstream of the transcriptional start site are several other sequences recognized by cellular factors. Leader binding protein (LBP-1)/ untranslated binding protein-1 (UBP-1) recognizes two sites: one high affinity site which extends from -16 to +27, and one low affinity site from -38 to -16.[540] In vitro transcriptional studies would suggest UBP-1/LBP-1, a 63 kilodalton protein, can bind the low affinity site in the LTR and modestly inhibit transcription by blocking access to the general transcriptional factor TFIID; but only if incubated with the target DNA prior to addition of TFIID.[424,497,541] This would suggest that this protein could participate in the level of transcriptional initiation from the HIV-1-LTR.[424,497,541] CTF/NF-1 binds sequences from +40 to +45[424] and another factor termed untranslated binding protein-2 (UBP-2) appears to recognize nucleotides +28 to +36.[393] While it remains to be determined if any of these downstream sequences and their binding factors materially influence the level of viral gene expression in vivo, there is another sequence, *trans*-activation response region or TAR from nucleotides 14-45 which is critically important to the level of viral mRNA expression (discussed in detail above).

A unique feature of these retroviral agents that has received little attention and yet may be important to its pathogenesis is the presence of two copies of the long terminal repeat. While we have discussed in detail all of the potential cellular and viral derived proteins which interact with the 5'LTR, it must be remembered that an identical set of target DNA sequences exist at the 3' end of the integrated provirus, including the TAR region which might be expected to generate *tat* responsive nascent mRNAs. Klaver and Berkhout addressed this issue by creating full length plasmids which in addition, contained a chloramphenicol acetyltransferase (CAT) reporter gene driven by the 3'LTR.[542] They found that, indeed, both LTRs are *tat* responsive, but that the 5'LTR was dramatically more active than the 3'LTR. They could however, increase expression from the 3'LTR by inactivating the 5'LTR. In addition, somewhat surprisingly, they could dampen 5'LTR expression by increasing 3'LTR expression.[542] This phenomenon of promoter exclusion has been well described for simple retroviruses and a number of other cellular promoters.[543-547] One hypothesis offered to explain these events is that the continual RNA polymerase II trafficking downstream does not allow the effective interaction of the downstream promoter with its transcriptional factors.[542,546-548] While this could explain why the 3'LTR is less effectively used in the presence of an active 5'LTR, it does not explain why the 5'LTR would be inhibited in the presence of an active 3'LTR since the downstream trafficking of RNA polymerase II is traveling away from the 5'LTR. Another hypothesis offered is that there is competition for a limiting transcriptional factor and whichever LTR binds this factor is the one used. Arguing against this hypothesis is the lack of any inhibitory effect by transfection of excess LTRs into cells.[542,546-548] A third hypothesis is that there is a conformational change in the DNA topology which can be transmitted either downstream or upstream of whichever LTR is being used. This concept of DNA topology as a determinant of promoter activity is discussed more fully in chapter 3. It is likely that this is the operative mechanism of the promoter exclusion demonstrated by Klaver and Berkhout.[542] This still leaves open the question of how a cell decides which of the integrated proviral LTRs to target for binding

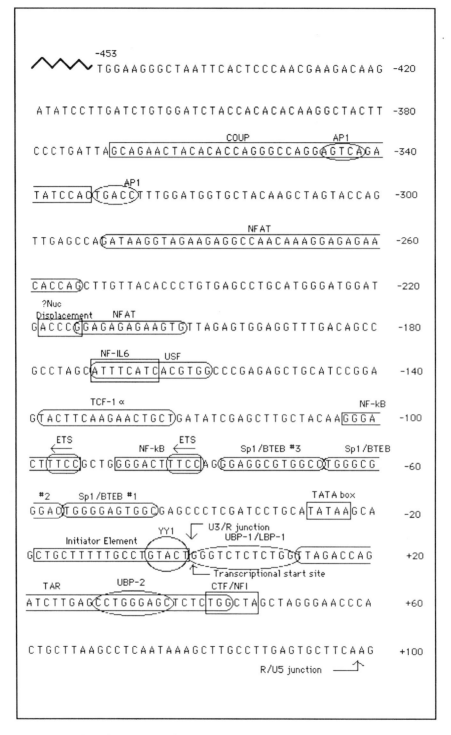

Fig. 2.12. Nucleotide sequence of HIV-1 LTR with overlying binding factors. As discussed in the text, there are multiple potential binding sites for cellular factors within the U3/R region of the LTR. While clearly some of these factors are critical to determining the transcriptional state of the LTR, the functional significance of many of these factors remains to be determined. (Adapted from Gaynor R. AIDS 1992; 6:347-363.)

of the many transcriptional factors outlined above. There are preliminary data to suggest that the 3'LTR has a different DNase I hypersensitivity pattern (suggesting a different pattern of DNA sequence usage) when compared with the 5'LTR.[383] What is not clear under these
circumstances is which pattern of DNase I protection reflects promoter
activity versus inactivity. One retrovirally determined explanation for
the preferential usage of the 5'LTR could lie in the intragenic enhancer sequences which have been reported.[381-383,549-550] If these elements
are position dependent they might effect one LTR in preference over
the other.[542] At least one study reports the presence of a fusion gene
product originating from the 3'LTR.[551] In a similar vein, a number of
explanations have been offered as to why only the 3'LTR polyadenylation
signal (AAUAAA) appears to be used with any frequency despite an
identical copy present in the 5'LTR.[552-557]

CO-PATHOGENS AND HIV-1 GENE EXPRESSION

One consequence of the attempts to define the pathogenesis of
HIV-1 infection was the search for co-pathogens. While a number of
scenarios exist inter-relating other infectious pathogens to the progression of disease, we will confine our discussion to those agents that
directly interact with the HIV-1 provirus and effect its level of transcription by elaborating transcriptional factors. An early group of agents
nominated as co-pathogens in HIV-1 infection were members of the
herpes virus family.

Because of its clinical prevalence in the HIV-1 infected population, human cytomegalovirus (HCMV) has received a great deal of
attention. An obvious confinement imposed by the requirement for
direct interaction between pathogens is the necessity for dual infection
of a single cell. There have, in fact, been a number of reports demonstrating such dual infection with HIV-1 and HCMV, although they
have largely been confined to cells of the central nervous system.[558-561]
There have been, in general, two approaches to assess the impact of
HCMV infection on expression of genes from the HIV-1 LTR: (i) use
of isolated transcriptional proteins from HCMV in the presence of
HIV-1 and (ii) dual infection of cells with whole virus and the consequent measurement of viral output from both viruses. Several laboratories have taken the first approach and identified gene products of
HCMV capable of transactivating the HIV-1 LTR.[562-565] The immediate early genes of HCMV have significant *trans*-regulatory potential in
control of the HCMV life cycle and have therefore received the majority of attention in terms of their effect on HIV-1 expression.
The protein products of the immediate early HCMV genes are complicated, arising from multiple exons and yielding various isoforms
depending upon splicing patterns.[566-568] Three of these isoforms IE55,
IE72, and IE86, were extensively investigated by Ghazal et al who
demonstrated a complicated pattern of transactivation of the HIV-1
LTR.[569] They demonstrated that there is a critical 155 amino acid
region of IE86 which was required for the synergistic transactivation
of the LTR by IE72. Furthermore, they implicated an additional cellular
protein in this transactivation. Mutational analysis of the target LTR

mapped this *synergistic* response region to position -174 to -163, which overlaps the USF region.[569] It is interesting that HCMV genes which also respond synergistically to IE72 and IE86, contain a potential USF binding site within one of its promoters.[568,570]

While the USF sequences have been firmly established as the target for the synergy between IE72 and IE86, surprisingly, the precise sequences responsible for each individual immediate early gene products' transactivation has remained obscure.[569] Barry et al initially reported that the initiator region (-6 to +20) of the LTR to be responsible for the HCMV immediate early gene response; however, other studies have failed to define such a circumscribed response element.[562,563,565,571] The demonstration that IE72 may function to transactivate HCMV genes by induction of NF-κB has complicated these studies by the potential for multiple effects of these gene products.[572] To better define the role of NF-κB in the IE72 response, Gaynor et al evaluated the effects of NF-κB target site mutations on response of the HIV-1 LTR to IE72 and IE86.[573] While there was a somewhat lower level of transcription at baseline (as expected) with these mutants, they remained responsive to both of these HCMV gene products suggesting that NF-κB was at least not the sole mechanism of transactivation in response to IE72.[573]

Given the complex (and sometimes contradictory) effects of individual HCMV gene products on HIV-1 expression, it is not surprising that the study of whole virus interactions has yielded a wide range of effects on HIV-1 expression from stimulatory, to neutral, to inhibitory.[574-577] Because the majority of studies on dually infected cells have suggested that the cells most at risk for co-habitation with HCMV and HIV-1 reside within the central nervous system, cell lines derived from this source have been widely used.[558,560,561] A recent large study has identified three patterns of interaction between HCMV and HIV-1 in central nervous system derived cells.[578] In cells fully permissive for both HCMV and HIV-1, there appeared to be an inhibitory effect on HIV-1 gene expression in the presence of both viruses. In cells in which HCMV expression is restricted but HIV-1 is permissive, there is no effect on HIV-1 gene expression. The cell line SY5Y (HCMV permissive) fails to support HIV-1 expression when infected alone, however, transiently supports a high level HIV-1 replication when co-infected with HCMV.[578] Given the individual complexity of gene expression of each of these viruses, these findings lend themselves to multiple interpretations. It is tempting to speculate that in cells which are dually permissive for HIV-1 and HCMV, there is competition for some limiting cellular factor that results in HIV-1's down-regulation. One immediate candidate for such a factor is USF which is apparently utilized in the transcriptional regulation of both viruses. The fact that in cells which fail to express HCMV, there is no effect on HIV-1 expression in the presence of both viruses merely demonstrates that there are potential interactions between these agents under the right circumstances. Similarly, the finding that SY5Y cells can transiently overcome their restriction to expression of HIV-1 gene products in the presence of actively expressed HCMV viral gene products further substantiates these interactions.

While the study of these interactions between HCMV *trans*-regulatory gene products with the HIV-1 LTR is of intellectual interest and may offer insights into the many components contributing to the control of HIV-1 expression, the overall contribution to the level of circulating virus in the patient remains unknown. One could speculate that there is some participation of dually infected cells in the pathogenic process given the potential overlap in host range of HCMV and HIV-1 within macrophages of the central nervous system. Similarly, while the interaction of the adenovirus E1A transcriptional factor with the HIV-1 LTR has contributed significantly to our understanding of HIV-1's transcriptional control mechanisms (particularly in comparison with *tat*'s transactivation), the clinical significance of dual infections with HIV-1 and adenoviruses remains to be established.[578,580]

Another herpes virus to draw attention to its effects on HIV-1 expression is herpes simplex virus type 1 (HSV1). Two HSV1 immediate early viral gene products, ICP0 and ICP4, have been identified in transient expression systems to increase HIV-1 LTR driven gene expression.[581-584] Similar to the HCMV immediate early gene products, the precise targets within the LTR for the action of ICP0 and ICP4 have defied identification.[585] Interestingly, overexpression of these individual genes in cells containing an integrated HIV-1 LTR fails to result in transactivation.[585] In contrast, whole virus infection can effectively lead to increased HIV-1 replication from an integrated provirus.[586] Activation by HSV1 whole virus infection results in the binding of proteins of 55 kilodalton and 85 dilodalton to the NF-κB sites; and also leads to binding of a 50 kilodalton protein, termed HLP-1, to the LBP-1 site.[586-588] Attempts to unravel the mechanism of HSV1's transactivation of HIV1 have employed acyclovir, an inhibitor of HSV1 replication.[585] While blocking late gene expression, acyclovir does not block expression of either the immediate early genes or early genes of HSV1. Since the immediate early genes have been implicated in the transactivation of the HIV-1 virus, it was not surprising that acyclovir did not block HSV1's ability to activate HIV-1 expression in ACH-2 cells; what was somewhat surprising however, was that acyclovir inhibited the binding of the 55 and 85 kilodalton proteins to the NF-κB site and the binding of HLP-1 to the LBP-1 site.[585] Furthermore, in this study, ICP0 but not ICP4, increased viral expression from ACH-2 cells. These authors speculate that ICP0 acts cooperatively with NF-κB and HLP-1 to achieve transcriptional activation; and despite the lower levels of NF-κB and HLP-1, in absence of late HSV-1 gene expression, there are still sufficient numbers of these molecules for interaction with ICP0 to achieve viral activation.[585] As with HCMV, there is no clear consensus on the mechanism of HSV1's activation of the HIV-1 LTR. Furthermore, as with HCMV, there is, in all likelihood, little opportunity for these viruses to interact to a significant degree in vivo except perhaps through elaboration of cytokines.

One herpes virus which has a greater likelihood of finding itself in the same cell with HIV-1 is human herpes virus 6 (HHV6). HHV6 infects lymphocytes, including CD4+ lymphocytes; moreover, it has been demonstrated that infection of CD8+ lymphocytes by HHV6 induces surface expression of the CD4 molecule and might thereby increase the susceptibility of CD8+ cells to HIV-1 infection.[589,590] There are conflicting reports, however, on HHV6's effect on HIV-1 expression. Levy et al and Carrigan et al report suppression of HIV-1 replication by simultaneous infection with HHV6.[591,592] In contrast, Ensoli et al report transactivation of the HIV-1 LTR by HHV6 through a core enhancer dependent mechanism.[593] Wang et al similarly find that a genomic fragment of HHV6 (ZVH14) can transactivate the HIV-1 LTR but they demonstrate a dependence on Sp-1 binding sites.[594,595] Luso et al have demonstrated increased cytopathicity in CD4 positive cells dually infected with HIV-1 and HHV6.[589] Given the very high seroprevalence to HHV6 within the general population, it could theoretically have a clinical impact on HIV-1 expression; however, no such role has been established to date.

RETROVIRAL LATENCY

To summarize, we would propose from the virologic point of view that there are potentially two early levels of restriction to HIV-1 gene expression, one determined at the level of viral transcriptional initiation which is influenced by a number of cellular DNA -binding factors (i.e. NF-κB, Sp-1, Ap-1, LBP-1, CTF/NF-1, URS, USF, COUP, YY1) which interact with the HIV-1 LTR. While the relative influence of each of these factors remains to be defined exactly (and may depend upon the specific tissue), the role of NF-κB is central to the overall level of initiation of HIV-1 transcripts. In addition to this control over viral transcriptional initiation, there is a threshold effect in which the levels of the HIV-1 regulatory proteins derived from multiply-spliced mRNA determine the fate of initiated viral transcripts to promote more efficient elongation of initiated mRNA (*Tat*) and to prevent the splicing of these transcripts (*Rev*); this in turn promotes the translation of viral structural proteins and full length genomic templates for packaging into viral particles. A third level of restriction or latency not considered in this discussion is the control of viral assembly and release which may be mediated by the some of the other regulatory proteins derived from the viral genome.

HYPOTHETICAL MODEL OF HIV-1 PATHOGENESIS

After the initial exposure to a small level of inoculating virus, a few cells become productively infected leading to a large viremia in the window period prior to establishment of an immune response. As a result of the remarkably high affinity of HIV-1 gp120 surface glycoprotein for the CD4 molecule, this plasma viremia leads to a large number of CD4 positive cells being infected during this non-immune phase of infection. With the induction of HIV-1 specific cytoxic T cells there is clearance of infected cells which are actively producing viral antigens and a marked reduction in plasma viremia. Following the production of these cytotoxic T cells, there is left a large number of cells which have integrated HIV-1 provirus but which are not actively expressing viral antigens and therefore escape immune destruction. A portion of these cells do not express viral antigens because they have a defective provirus lacking in a functional *tat* or *rev* protein or deletion of some other vital portion of the viral genome.[596] Another portion of cells have a fully functional virus which is maintained in a latent state either from a lack of necessary transcriptional factors (in the quiescent state) or as a result of the random site of integration (see chapter 3). During the ensuing 10-15 years, as a result of either T-cell:macrophage interaction during the course of normal immunologic challenges or local cytokine production, a certain portion of these latently infected cells undergo a physiological change resulting in active production of virus. Only a small minority of cells undergo such a physiological change at any given time accounting for the large percentage of proviral positive cells remaining transcriptionally silent throughout the course of infection. Each of the few cells which *do* undergo a change in transcriptional activity (which eventually leads to their immune destruction) generates a large number of viral particles which provide the substrate for the low fidelity reverse transcriptase enzyme and lead to new rounds of proviral integration. A significant proportion of these *newly* infected cells will express viral antigens that lead to their elimination (and the continual taxation on CD4+ lymphocyte reserves). The remaining proportion of newly infected cells will be latently infected as with the initial round of infection; *and* a tiny minority of these will have attained a mutation leading to an altered epitope providing a temporary (or even perhaps permanent) selective advantage. Alternatively, these mutations may lead to a drifting phenotype toward a more cytopathic variant[597-601] (i.e. synctium inducing variants). During the 10-15 years of smoldering infection, there is ultimately selection and amplification of viral variants which escape the fatiguing immune system and as the host moves closer to the clinically symptomatic stages, there is less and less efficient elimination of cells actively producing virus. This leads to even higher rates of virus production with ever more integrative events leading to active virus production and low fidelity reverse transcription with generation of ever more mutants; and finally the overwhelming of CD4+ cells with their rapid decline and onset of symptomatic disease heralded by opportunistic infections.

While there is much of this model which remains speculative (and bleak), it holds a number of points at which clinical intervention might prove successful in this complex host-virus interaction. One such point is the early identification of infected patients with aggressive institution of antiviral therapy aimed at multiple points in the viral life cycle. In addition to reverse transcriptase inhibitors, two particularly promising targets for intervention are the *tat* and *rev* proteins which are so critical in determining the level of effective transcription from the HIV-1 provirus. A number of clinical strategies have already been undertaken in this regard. Additional clinical interventions might include attempts at gentle immune suppression early in infection to prevent the intermittent reactivation cycles which provide the substrate for generation of mutant virus; or prevention of chromatin re-organization which is predicted to precede reactivation of those proviruses whose latency is determined by integration site. Given the permanence of the integrative event in most circumstances and the relatively long life expectancy of the cells involved, HIV-1 infection will not likely be truly curable anytime in the near future. In the interim, we are left to attempt extension of the clinical latency period by intervention in as many of these transcriptional regulatory steps as possible, while walking the fine line between transcriptional suppression of HIV-1 without suppression of vital cellular genes.

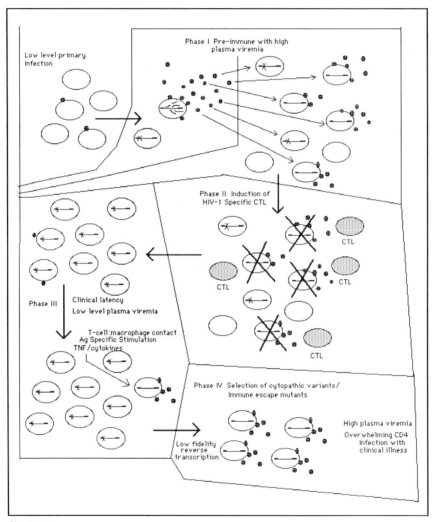

Fig. 2.13A

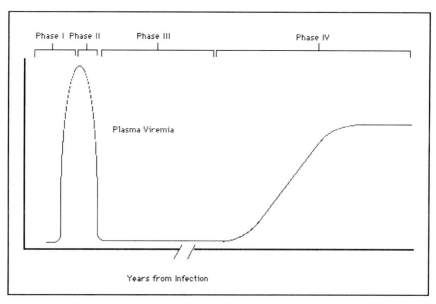

Fig. 2.13B

Figs. 2.13A and 2.13B. Hypothetical model of the pathogenesis of HIV-1 infection. In Phase I, there is the introduction of a minimal level of inoculating virus into the host which results in a small number of cells being infected. Some of the newly infected cells actively produce virus while others remain transcriptionally silent either as a result of integration site, or lack of necessary transcriptional factor within the cell (i.e. quiescent T cells), or acquisition of a "fatal" mutation during reverse transcription. The few cells which are transcriptionally active are free to produce large numbers of virus unimpeded by the immune system. This leads to an initial high plasma viremia (panel B, above) and infection of a large number of cells (panel A, opposite page). In Phase II, there is induction of HIV-1 specific cytotoxic T lymphocytes and a subsequent clearing of cells actively producing virus (panel A, opposite page) and a sharp reduction of plasma viremia (panel B, above). In Phase III, there are a very small number of cells which "leak" small amounts of virus but the majority of cells remain transcriptionally silent under the selective pressure of the immune system. A minority of cells at any given time can re-activate viral production in response to an antigen specific stimulus or in response to locally produced cytokines with a brief "burst" of virus production leading to additional round of infection, subject to low fidelity reverse transcription and the generation of mutants (panel A, opposite page). It would also be predicted that this re-activated cell would then be targeted for immune destruction. While on an organismal level there is probably never a truly latent period, the level of circulating virus is exceptionally low (panel B, above). In phase IV, after many years of these repeated cycles, there is outgrowth of immune escape mutants or generation of rapidly cytopathic viral variants which overwhelm the already taxed CD4+ lymphocyte pool; and consequently there is marked immune dysfunction leading ultimately to opportunistic infection and death.

CHAPTER 3

HOST DETERMINANTS OF RETROVIRAL GENE EXPRESSION

OVERVIEW

A great deal of attention has been devoted to the fine detail of individual retroviruses. The ready access of most laboratories to sequencing technologies has allowed the nucleotide by nucleotide comparison of many different retroviruses providing many insights into the mechanism of proviral gene regulation. As detailed elsewhere in this text, many of the basic proviral regulatory sequences have been identified, most of which are not unique to retroviruses but are shared among many eukaryotic genes. Similarly, the fine detail of eukaryctic gene expression has yielded significant insight into the protein:DNA interactions required for efficient transcription. The description of nuclear factor *kappa* B (NF-κB) isolated from B cells in the mid 1980s proved to be a particularly illustrative study of such an interaction.[438] NF-κB was shown to be quickly inducible in B cells; to subsequently migrate to the nucleus where it bound a specific 11 base pair sequence within the promoter/enhancer of the kappa chain of immunoglobulin; and to result in the up-regulation of antibody production. This induction of NF-κB was initially held to explain tissue specific gene expression.[438] As more and more genes were analyzed, however, it became clear that many genes share sequence specific *cis* elements within their enhancers. One notable example of such shared use of sequence specific transcriptional factors is, in fact, the NF-κB family of proteins. There are now multiple cellular and viral genes identified which use NF-κB (or members of the related *rel*-family of oncoproteins) as inducible transcriptional factors, including HIV-1, HIV-2, SIV, MHC II, IL-2, β-2 microglobulin, β-IFN, Ig kappa enhancer, serum amyloid A, urokinse and even the p50 subunit of NF-κB itself.[421,439,441-442,491-495] This obviously necessitates additional levels of transcriptional control beyond primary sequences and cognate binding protein(s) for transcriptional control of tissue specific genes.

Since a key feature of all retroviral life cycles is integration into the host cell's genome it might be expected that this small viral gene cluster (now placed in the context of the surrounding genome) might fall under the same transcriptional influences as native genes, the majority of which remain unexpressed. One of the most significant regulatory elements within the SIV, HIV-1 and HIV-2 promoter/enhancer is, in fact, NF-κB. As suggested above, there must be mechanisms which regulate the response of individual genes to induction of NF-κB since each somatic cell within an organism contains the genetic information to express all of the NF-κB driven genes and yet within any given tissue type only a minority (if any) of these genes are expressed. An examination of the mechanism(s) whereby a cell differentially expresses NF-κB driven genes in the presence of this transcriptional factor may provide insight into the mechanism(s) of proviral latency. Mechanisms postulated to contribute to this differential gene expression are tissue specific assembly of genes into higher order chromatin structures such as nucleosomes, and chromatin loops (or domains) which are bounded by matrix attachment regions. Since randomly integrated proviral sequences find themselves within this environment it is essential to examine these potential host influences on retroviral gene expression. To accomplish this, a knowledge of the basic units of chromatin organization is required. We will review below the accumulated data on the regulation of both eukaryotic and viral gene expression by higher order chromatin structures.

NUCLEOSOMES AND TRANSCRIPTIONAL POTENTIAL

Cellular genomic DNA, over the vast majority of its length, is tightly complexed with cellular proteins. The most abundant (and highly conserved) of these DNA binding proteins are histones. There are six highly basic proteins within the histone family designated: H1, H2A, H2B, H3, H4 and H5. The simplest unit of organization of chromatin is the nucleosome which consists of an octamer of histones, comprised of two each of H2A, H2B, H3 and H4 around which is wrapped approximately 145-150 base pairs of DNA. Between individual nucleosomes are approximately 50-55 base pairs of DNA which allow the flexibility for further compaction into the 30 nm fiber. Histone H1 or H5 associates with the neighboring nucleosomes where it serves to stabilize chromatin in this highly compact configuration (reviewed in refs. 604,605). These relationships are illustrated in Figure 3.14.

Nucleosome assembly over specific genes and their regulatory elements have been shown to influence a number of transcriptional systems.[606-613] While there is general acceptance that actively transcribed regions of chromatin are in a less condensed configuration, allowing for greater access to transcriptional protein complexes[616,617] the exact nature and specificity of the nucleosomal mediated modification of transcription is only now being unravelled.[618,619] One of the early findings to suggest that histones participated in the control of transcription was the failure of purified sequence specific transcriptional factors to significantly up-regulate transcription in in vitro transcription systems.[618] Only when the template DNA was pre-incubated with crude cellular extracts, including individual histones, did the transcriptional factors up-regulate transcription. It was subsequently shown that the initial failure of these factors to stimulate transcription was the high basal level of gene expression in the absence of assembly of template DNA into chromatin structures. It was widely held from this observation that histones had a generally repressive effect on gene expression while sequence specific transcriptional factors did something to relieve that repression.[618,619]

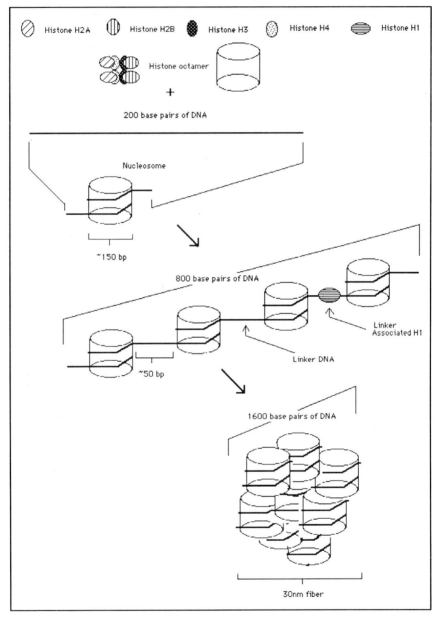

Fig. 3.14. Higher order chromatin organization. A cylindrical octamer of histones forms the basic structural unit of chromatin organization. Genomic DNA is wrapped approximately 1.75 times around this cylinder over a length of ~150 base pairs comprising the nucleosome. There are approximately 50 base pairs of linker DNA between nucleosomes which is generally occupied by a single molecule of H1. In transcriptionally incompetent, highly condensed chromatin, individual nucleosomes are ordered into the 30 nm chromatin fiber which effectively denies access to the transcriptional protein complex.

One mechanism widely held to contribute to this effect is the physical obstruction of sequence specific transcriptional factors from their cognate binding sites by assembly of the DNA into nucleosomes. Indeed, a body of evidence suggests that nucleosomes compete with transcriptional pre-initiation complexes for binding of sequence specific regions within regulatory elements.[609,612,622-627] Matsui and Workman et al independently showed in 1987 that the major late promoter of adenovirus was transcriptionally silent when reconstituted into chromatin in vitro if the transcriptional factors were added *after* reconstitution.[624,625] If, however, the transcriptional factors were pre-incubated with the target DNA prior to reconstitution, transcription was active. Furthermore it was demonstrated that the TATA binding protein, TFIID, was sufficient for maintaining the promoter in a potentially responsive configuration.[625] If the isolated TFIID factor was pre-incubated with target DNA prior to chromatin reconstitution there was no active transcription. However, if now the other minimal transcriptional proteins were added transcription was fully active. Early work with the HIV-1 promoter in a chromatin assembly assay using purified TFIID and

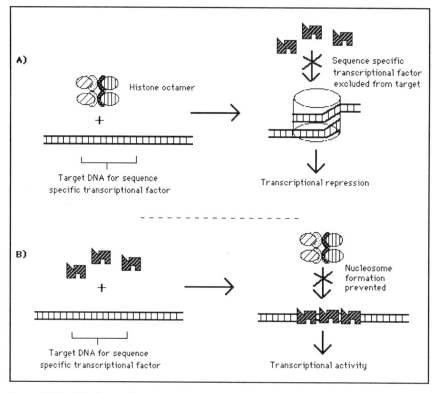

Fig. 3.15. Model of transcriptional factor competition for occupancy of sequence specific binding sites. In panel A, in vitro reconstitution of DNA target sequences within nucleosome structures prevent the subsequently added sequence specific transcriptional factor from gaining access to its target DNA with the consequent transcriptional repression. If, as depicted in panel B, the sequence specific transcriptional factors are allowed to bind prior to reconstitution into nucleosomes, histone condensation onto DNA is blocked with consequent transcriptional activity.

purified Sp-1 demonstrated the same principle of activation of transcription.[628] These observations were consistent with the model that binding of TFIID competes with histones for its target sequences within the viral promoter.

In similar studies using the 5S rRNA gene of *Xenopus*, Shimamura et al showed that reconstitution of target DNA into high density nucleosomes repressed transcription even in the absence of histone H1, while low density nucleosome reconstitution allowed transcription in the absence of histone H1 but not in its presence.[629] If, however, the sequence specific transcriptional factors were pre-incubated with target DNA, full transcriptional activity was achieved even in the presence of high density nucleosomes and histone H1.[629] Finally, Workman et al showed that transactivation by the pseudorabies virus immediate early protein functions by facilitating the binding of TFIID to its target.[625] Of note, is the demonstration by Yuan et al that this same pseudorabies virus gene product transactivated the HIV-1 and HIV-2 LTR; and that the effect was mapped by deletion mutation analysis to the region of the LTR containing the TATA box.[630] It is tantalizing to speculate that the transactivation of the HIV-1 and HIV-2 LTR by this pseudorabies virus immediate early protein is mediated through disruption of the histone:DNA interaction around the TATA box allowing freer access to this transcriptional factor, which in turn increases the transcriptional potential of these retroviruses.

Other evidence suggests that nucleosomes may function in certain transcriptional systems by preventing the efficient elongation of mRNA once transcriptional initiation has occurred, leading to premature termination of the nascent RNA transcript.[215] Transcriptional control of heat shock protein (hsp70) gene by environmental stress in *Drosophila melanogaster* has been the object of extensive investigation. A number of investigators have shown that in the uninduced state, the hsp70 structural gene is relatively resistant to nuclease digestion suggesting organization into compact nucleosomal structures.[631-634] Upon induction by environmental stress, this gene becomes nuclease susceptible. Unlike other transcriptional systems however, the promoter region of hsp70 remains nucleosome free even in the uninduced state. In addition, Rougive and Lis demonstrated that the heat shock transcriptional factor was bound to its target sequence within the promoter in the uninduced state and that there were even nascent RNA transcripts being made.[215] Only upon induction however did the nascent RNA transcripts elongate to full length messages for subsequent translation. At least one explanation for control of this gene complex (which requires rapid response times) is that the transcriptional machinery remains engaged in the nucleosome free promoter; and upon induction, there is relief of downstream obstructions such as nucleosomes which now allow efficient RNA polymerase readthrough.

Still other evidence suggests that nucleosome formation *augments* in vitro transcription when compared with naked DNA.[635-637] Contrary to the majority of transcriptional systems where nucleosome formation markedly decreases transcriptional rates, in the estrogen responsive vitellogenin B1 gene of *Xenopus*, chromatin reconstitution results in augmented transcription.[635] A potential explanation for this aberrant finding comes from the work of Schild et al who show that in the vitellogenin B1 promoter there is a precisely positioned nucleosome occupying nucleotides -140 to -300 relative to the transcriptional start site. If the positioning of this nucleosome was prevented by removal of these sequences, there was loss of estrogen responsiveness.[636] It is proposed that there is creation of a loop resulting from DNA wrapping around this nucleosome which brings the estrogen binding site of the enhancer in close proximity to the pre-initiation complexes assembled on the promoter.[637] This model has been previously proposed by Elgin as one explanation of how an enhancer which is placed far upstream can influence transcriptional initiation from the downstream promoter.[638] An alternative explanation is a requirement of the estrogen responsive target sequence to be configured into the context of a nucleosome for effective interaction. Precedent for such a requirement is found with the mouse mammary tumor virus's hormone responsive element.[639,640]

As more and more is learned of the effects of chromatin structure on the regulation of eukaryotic gene expression, it is clear that any consideration of integrated retroviral gene expression must include these mitigating influences. Unless there are elements within the retroviral promoter which allow escape from these influences (and to date no such element for any retorvirus has been described), it might be expected that the integrated provirus is incorporated into chromatin structures (such as nucleosomes); and that these structures influence transcriptional potential. Nucleosomal phasing has in fact been described for the mouse mammary tumor virus (MMTV) and for HIV-1 as discussed below.

NUCLEOSOMAL ORGANIZATION AND RETROVIRAL LTRs

Mouse Mammary Tumor Virus

Few transcriptional control systems have received as much attention as that of the mouse mammary tumor virus (MMTV). From this scrutiny has come the clear appreciation of the impact of chromatin structures on retroviral gene expression. DNA binding studies and linker-scanning mutational analysis clearly identified nuclear factor 1 (NF1) as an important sequence specific transcriptional factor for gene expression from the MMTV LTR.[641-644] In addition, the MMTV LTR is a classic steroid responsive promoter. An early assumption in the study of transcriptional regulation of this virus was that steroid treatment of infected cells would lead to an increase in NF1 with subsequent transcriptional stimulation. This assumption soon fell in the face of data showing that there was no significant increase in NF1 the presence of steroid treatment; and that protein synthesis was not required for the steroid effect on transcription to be seen.[642-644] By contrast, in the context of chromatin, it *was* demonstrated that NF1 was bound to its cognate sequence *only* in the presence of steroid treatment.[642] Since there was no difference in binding affinity of NF1 from steroid treated or untreated cells on *naked* DNA, it was suggested that steroid treatment resulted in some alteration in chromatin structure which led to binding of NF1 to it target sequence.[642]

Sequence specificity of nucleosomal binding was soon demonstrated both in vivo and in vitro in an MMTV LTR-CAT construct incorporated into a bovine papilloma virus (BPV) minichromosome.[645-647] Furthermore, in vitro reconstitution of nucleosomes using only small fragments of the BPV-based minichromosome revealed the same sequence specific positioning of the nucleosome over the steroid responsive region of the MMTV LTR as occurs in situ, suggesting that the information for positioning is contained within the LTR of this retrovirus.[647] There are six precisely positioned nucleosomes overlying the MMTV LTR as shown in Figure 3.16. As depicted, nucleosome B overlies the glucocorticoid responsive element (GRE) as well as the binding site for NF1. Pina et al showed that once the steroid receptor complex is transported to the nucleus, this specific nucleosome is modified to induce a nuclease hypersensitive site, implying greater access to this previously protected region of DNA. Surprisingly, the *specificity* of the glucocorticoid/receptor complex for its target sequence is 60- to 70-fold *higher* when incorporated into a nucleosome compared with its *specificity* of binding in naked DNA.[639] Furthermore, the binding affinity of the glucocorticoid-receptor complex to its cognate sequence incorporated into a nucleosome is influenced by translational positioning within the nucleosome.[640] This chromatin influence is however only present in stably maintained DNA. If the MMTV LTR is transiently introduced, the binding of NF1 and OCT proteins are constitutive and hormone independent.[648]

Finally, a great deal of attention has been paid to transcriptional initiation with considerably less attention paid to transcriptional repression. This issue has recently been addressed with the MMTV LTR driven transcription. Lee et al have shown that the hormone initiated transcription from this promoter is maximal within the first few hours of exposure to hormone; however, after 24 hours, transcription has returned to baseline despite the continued presence of steroid hormone.[649] Concomitant with this return to a basal level of transcription is the loss of the hypersensitivity site initially introduced (indicating the reformation of nucleosome B) and loss of NF1 binding. This effect is seen only in the stably maintained MMTV LTR and not seen with transiently introduced plasmids. The mechanism to re-establish this nucleosome is still speculative. One possibility was that the cell simply lacked the general transcriptional factors necessary for continued expression from this promoter. This was shown not to be the case by the demonstration that within these same cells, transiently introduced MMTV LTR constructs still maintained high levels of transcription suggesting no such shortage of these transcriptional factors. Another possibility which has some support from the yeast GAL gene expression system is that DNA replication contributes to re-establishment of the repressed chromatin configuration by creating another round of competition between histone deposition and transcriptional factor binding to DNA.[650] Almouzni and Wolffe showed that for maximal repression of basal levels of transcription from the GAL genes, nucleosome formation needed to occur in the context of DNA replication.[650] This seems unlikely to be the mechanism operative here however, since this repression of GAL gene expression was circumvented in the presence of the GAL sequence specific transcriptional factor; and with the MMTV LTR, maintaining hormone-receptor complexes within the cell did not prevent the transcriptional down-regulation. These observations have led to the speculation that another cellular factor is participating in the original dissolution of nucleosome B in response to hormone treatment (in conjunction with binding of the hormone:receptor complex to its target sequence incorporated into the nucleosome); and it is this factor which is exhausted with prolonged hormone exposure. While data does not exist to establish this hypothesis, the SWI family of proteins have been shown to be essential yeast proteins in the hormone:receptor induction pathway which results in chromatin reorganization.[651] These proteins are obvious candidate proteins for such a speculation.

Despite the remaining questions, this retroviral transcriptional system has provided an excellent model of chromatin's role in mitigating retroviral gene expression. The overall sequence of events in the induction of MMTV gene expression and subsequent down-regulation are depicted in Figure 3.16. Under baseline conditions, stably integrated MMTV has six precisely positioned nucleosomes overlying its LTR. Upon hormone induction, the hormone:receptor complex is transported to the nucleus where is specifically binds to its target sequence incorporated within nucleosome B. This binding, by unknown mechanisms, leads to dissolution of this nucleosome which now allows the efficient binding of NF1 and OCT proteins to their targets; the assembly of the general transcriptional factors; and the subsequent high level of expression of viral gene products. In the continued presence of the hormone:receptor complex there is a refractory period entered which is accompanied by re-formation of nucleosome B and loss of NF1/OCT binding.[639-644,648-650,652]

HIV-1 LTR
Verdin et al has conducted similar studies with the HIV-1 LTR in the context of the cellular genome in the latently infected cell lines U1 and ACH-2.[653] ACH-2 cells are derived from a chronically HIV-1 infected CEM cell line (T-lymphocyte in origin) which has been shown to produce minimal levels of virus.[654] The macrophage-like U1 cell line is similarly derived from chronically infected U937 cells.[122] Both cell lines can be stimulated ~100-fold to produce full length viral transcripts in the presence of a number of different cytokines. Microccocal nuclease and DNase I digestion patterns establish a precise positioning of nucleosomes over the HIV-1 LTR as shown in Figure 3.17.[653] Interestingly, after the three normally phased upstream nucleosomes, there is a nucleosome free region extending over much of the U3 region of the LTR. There is then a positioned nucleosome over the R-U5 region including the transcriptional start site. As discussed at length in chapter 2, the majority of the promoter/enhancer activity of the

LTR lies within this nucleosome free region. Beyond nucleosome 1 there is an extended linker region of approximately 125 base pairs followed by three normally phased nucleosomes.[653] This overall pattern of nucleosome phasing would suggest that the sequence specific transcriptional factors NF-κB and Sp-1 proteins have ready access to their target sequences. Upon induction of transcription with phorbol esters or tumor necrosis factor-α, there is creation of a nuclease hypersensitivity site over the nucleosome 1 position suggesting alteration of this structure into a more accessible configuration.[653] Of greater interest is

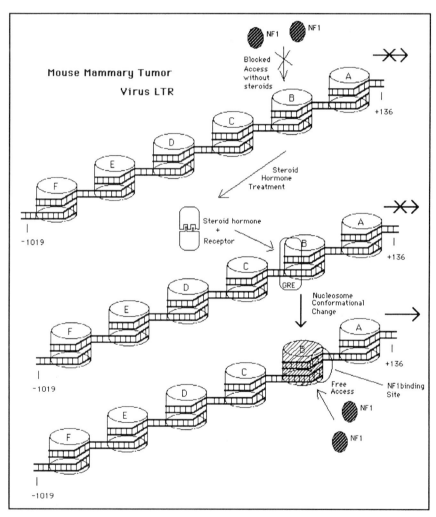

Fig. 3.16. Schematic representation of the transcriptional activation of the Mouse Mammary Tumor Virus (MMTV) LTR. There are six precisely positioned nucleosomes overlying the MMTV LTR. Nucleosome B incorporates the glucocorticoid response element (GRE) and in fact contributes to the specificity of binding of the steroid hormone:receptor complex to this site. Prior to GRE binding, NF1 which is a sequence specific transactivator of the MMTV LTR is present but unable to bind its target site which also is incorporated into nucleosome B. There is nucleosomal reorganization upon GRE binding which now allows the effective interaction between NF1 and the NF1 binding site with subsequent transcriptional activation.

the demonstration that this disruption of nucleosome 1 was independent of active RNA polymerase II transcription. Verdin et al demonstrated creation of the hypersensitivity site over nucleosome 1 with
phorbol ester treatment even in the presence of α–amanitin, an RNA
polymerase II inhibitor.[653] While this represents a single investigation,
if other model systems of HIV-1 latency show similar nucleosomal
patterns, it suggests that induction of free NF-κB leads to conformational changes in chromatin nearly 100 base pairs downstream of its
DNA binding site; and that the limiting step in transcriptional initiation is not access of NF-κB to its target DNA but rather some interaction within the binding region of nucleosome 1. Exactly how this
might be accomplished remains unclear. At first glance this nucleosome pattern is similar to *hsp70* discussed above where the promoter
remains nucleosome free and the transcriptional machinery engaged;
upon induction by heat shock, there is disruption of the downstream
obstruction leading to efficient transcription. There are also similarities with the GAL transcriptional system as discussed below.

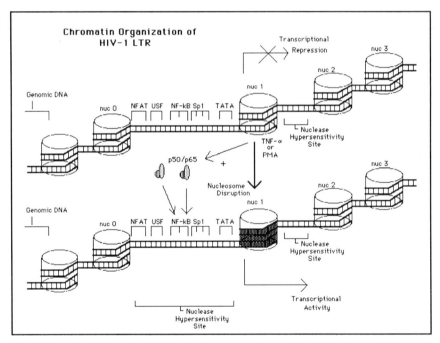

*Fig. 3.17. Chromatin organization of the HIV-1 Long Terminal Repeat. The HIV-1 LTR
maintains an extended nucleosome free region between nucleosome 0 and nucleosome 1. This region contains the essential enhancer/promoter sequences and these sites
may even be occupied with their respective transcriptional factors under baseline
conditions. Upon stimulation with either TNF-α or phorbol esters there is a conformational change within nucleosome 1 which creates a hypersensitivity site (even in the
absence of RNA polymerase II activity) and consequent transcriptional activation.[653] The
significance of the short nucleosome free region between nucleosome 1 and nucleosome
2 is unknown. As discussed in the text in chapter 2, one model for transcriptional
regulation of U1 cells is the continual generation of short promoter proximal transcripts
which fail to elongate. Upon conformational re-organization of nucleosome 1 it might be
speculated that the impediment to elongation is relieved and increased transcriptional
activity.*

YEAST PHO5 AND GAL GENE REGULATION

A somewhat clearer picture is emerging from the study of several yeast transcriptional systems. The promoter region of the acid phosphatase gene of yeast demonstrates sequence specific positioning of nucleosomes which become modified upon induction.[606,607,611,655-657] Yeast grown in the presence of low inorganic phosphate actively express the acid phosphatase gene while yeast grown in the presence of high inorganic phosphate repress it. Within the promoter region of the acid phosphatase gene are four upstream activating sequences (UAS).[606] Three of these four regions are specifically assembled into nucleosomes in the presence of high inorganic phosphate (repressed state) while all four are free of nucleosomes in the presence of low inorganic phosphate (expressed state).[607] Furthermore, if these cells are engineered to under-express histone H4 (and thereby disrupt nucleosome assembly) the acid phosphatase gene is fully expressed in the presence of either high or low inorganic phosphate.[655] In this relatively simple system, nucleosome assembly over the upstream activator sequences appear to prevent access of a transcriptional factor necessary for transcriptional initiation. Study of this transcriptional system has yielded another important insight into nucleosome regulation. Given the in vitro data where there is competition between transcriptional factors and nucleosomes for target sequences; and that pre-formed nucleosome structures prevented subsequent transcription in vitro it has been suggested that DNA replication is required to allow another round of competition between nucleosome deposition and pre-initiation complex formation which maintains the underlying DNA in a transcriptional competent configuration. Using a temperature sensitive mutant of the repressive PHO80 gene, Schmid et al were able to show that the positioned nucleosomes overlying the PHO5 promoter could be removed (in the absence of PHO80 expression) and subsequently reformed (in the presence of PHO80) without DNA replication.[658] The disruption of nucleosomes over the PHO5 promoter was glucose dependent (suggesting an energy requirement) while the re-formation was glucose independent.[658] This independence of nucleosome disruption on DNA replication was also suggested for MMTV and rat tyrosine aminotransferase induction by steroid hormones. In cells with doubling times in excess of 12 hours, it was demonstrated that chromatin re-organization took place in a matter of minutes.[649,659]

The other yeast transcriptional system which has yielded insight into nucleosome participation in gene regulation is the galactose responsive genes (GAL). Three major regulatory proteins control expression of this family of genes: GAL4, GAL80 and GAL3. The DNA binding protein, GAL4, acts through the upstream activating sequences (shared by all of these genes) to increase expression of the GAL1-10 structural genes when cells are grown in the presence of galactose (reviewed in ref. 660). GAL 80 acts to down-regulate the expression of these genes when cells are grown in non-galactose containing media and to temper the levels of expression in the presence of galactose; and is induced by an upstream activating sequence (UAS) which involves the same GAL4 protein. The chromatin organization of all of these genes are similar.[661,662] They contain a large nucleosome free region in the 5' portion of the promoter which contains the UAS flanked upstream by an array of nucleosomes and a positioned nucleosome downstream which covers the TATA box and trancsription start site. At first glance, this nucleosomal pattern is similar to that described for HIV-1 where the significant transcriptional factor binding sites are within a hypersensitive site with a positioned nucleosome overlying the transcriptional start site and three normally phased nucleosomes upstream of the hypersensitivity site. Unlike HIV-1 however, when GAL80 is induced, it is the upstream nucleosomes which are altered.[662]

Two additional features of the GAL gene regulatory system deserve attention in regard to chromatin's participation in gene expression. Fedor et al described a short sequence which partially overlaps one of the four UAS of the GAL promoter region which bound a factor (called factor Y).[521] This factor Y was shown to be responsible for maintaining the 230 base pair nucleosome free region characteristic of this promoter region. If this short sequence was placed in other backgrounds, it maintained a nucleosome free region. Chasman et al subsequently identified this 127,000 M.W. protein (renamed GRF2) and showed it to be a relatively abundant cellular protein with DNA binding sites in a number of cellular genes with the following consensus sequence: YNNNYYACCCG.[522] Given the overall similarity in nucleosomal phasing over the HIV-1 LTR it is of particular note that the HIV-1 LTR contains an ACCCG sequence within the 250 base pair nucleosome free region. It will be interesting to see if there is a homologous factor identified in U1 and ACH-2 cells which may function to circumvent condensation of the LTR within nucleosomes.

The second feature which this system has yielded is the recent independent demonstrations that the GAL4 protein can bind its target DNA within a nucleosome and that this binding (even in the absence of the activator domain of the protein) can cause nucleosome disruption.[663-665] Workman and Kingston further demonstrate that there is a transient complex formed between the target sequence incorporated into the nucleosome and the GAL4 protein. If naked competitor DNA is added to this complex, there is formation of either the nucleosome alone or GAL4:DNA complex alone and that the ternary complex of the three components is only an unstable intermediate on the way to the more stable complex of either GAL4:DNA or histone:DNA. Similar to the above data with the PHO5 gene, this chromatin re-organization in the presence of the GAL4 binding protein occurs in the absence of DNA replication.[650]

DYNAMICS OF CHROMATIN STRUCTURE

To allow for DNA replication and cell cycle specific transcription of genes, this condensation of DNA and histones into nucleosomes must be reversible.[666-669] Post-translational modifications of histones such as acetylation/deacetylation are major potential mechanisms for histones to rapidly change their affinity for DNA and thereby change chromosomal conformation.[616,670] Indeed, there is evidence that histones associated with actively transcribed (and less condensed) genes are more highly acetylated than histones associated with inactive areas of chromatin.[671,672] Analysis of bulk histones from activated lymphocytes show a higher percentage of acetylated forms compared with resting lymphocytes.[673] Additionally, site directed mutagenesis analysis of histone H4 mediated repression of the silent mating locus (HML) of *Saccharomyces cerevisiae* revealed a critical amino acid which is one of the amino acids involved in acetylation.[674,675] Substitution of the positively charged lysine at residue 16 (whose positive charge is neutralized by acetylation) by the neutral amino acid alanine resulted in derepression of this gene. Substitution of this lysine by another positively charged, non-acetylatable residue such as arginine maintained the repressed phenotype suggesting that post-translational charge modifications of histone H4 (such as by acetylation/deacetylation) may regulate expression of this gene.[674,675]

Sodium butyrate is a non-competitive histone deacetylase inhibitor that leads to the accumulation of hyperacetylated histones[521,676-680] and as such, has been used as a valuable tool to explore the effect of histone acetylation on individual gene expression. One of the attractive features of histone acetylation as a modulator of gene expression is the rapid turnover of acetyl groups. There appears to be at least two populations of histones in regard to acetylation, one in which the half life of acetyl groups is on the order of 3-15 minutes; the other groups has a half life on the order of 1-3 hours. The process of acetyl turnover is mediated by at least two different enzymes: one the histone acetyltransferase enzymes and the other the deacetylating enzyme(s). This hyperacetylation results in elongation of nucleosome structures, an increase in accessibility to intercalating agents, a decrease in thermal stability and a decrease in particle linking number reflecting the level of chromatin supercoiling.[678,682-684] Sodium butyrate has been shown to up-regulate a number of viral genes, including LTR-driven CAT expression in transiently transfected cells.[681,685-690] It has similarly been shown to modulate a number of cellular genes by increasing[680,691-695] (and in some cases decreasing[696,697] their expression. One example where sodium butyrate appeared to have a negative effect on transcription was, in fact, within the MMTV LTR system. It was shown that sodium butyrate treatment of cells with stably integrated MMTV constructs abolished their hormone responsiveness.[698] This finding remained largely inexplicable (within most models of action proposed for sodium butyrate) until the recent findings that nucleosomal organization of the hormone:receptor-target DNA in the MMTV LTR *increases* specificity of binding. It was widely held that hyperacetylation of core histones as a result of sodium butyrate treatment resulted in a less tightly associated nucleosome allowing greater access of transcriptional factors to the associated target DNA. One likely explanation for this finding is that the hyperacetylation resulting from sodium butyrate treatment modifies this nucleosome resulting in a less efficient interaction between the hormone:receptor complex and its target DNA. Loss of this interaction might then prevent the specific disruption of this nucleosome to allow access to NF1.

In contrast to the abolition of the hormone responsive effect in

MMTV gene expression, sodium butyrate has been shown by a number of investigators to significantly up-regulate expression from the HIV-1 LTR.[685-687,689,699] A number of attempts to define the exact sequences within the LTR responsible for the sodium butyrate response have led to conflicting results.[685,687,689] Using linker scanning mutants of the entire LTR, Laughlin et al were unable to define any region which significantly effected the sodium butyrate response.[685] In contrast, Bohan et al describe two regions, one immediately downstream of the NF-κB binding sites and another sequence after the transcriptional start site.[687] Golub reported yet another sequence, the TATA box, as essential to the sodium butyrate response.[699] In each case, the effects were mapped in the context of transient transfections which does not allow for stable integration of the gene of interest. As shown for the MMTV system, stable integration is required for the accurate assessment of chromatin's impact on transcription. To address the issue of stable integration, Laughlin et al demonstrated in a rhabdomyosarcoma derived cell line that a stably integrated LTR-CAT construct was significantly more responsive to sodium butyrate than a transiently transfected construct. In addition, they found that this stable cell line was not responsive to either phorbol esters (PMA) or tumor necrosis factor-α (TNF-α) alone, despite their efficient induction of free nuclear NF-κB.[700] Furthermore, sodium butyrate acted synergistically with either PMA or TNF-α. These data were taken to suggest that in this restricted transcriptional environment, two events were required for efficient transcription from the HIV-1 LTR: (i) a disruption of underlying repressive chromatin organization induced through histone hyperacetylation by sodium butyrate; and (ii) the induction of the sequence specific transcriptional factor NF-κB.

As evidenced above, one level of chromatin organization is compaction of DNA and histones into nucleosomes. The precise influence of this association on transcription is still being debated given the sometimes contradictory experimental results. Reconciliation of these discrepant results probably lies in the exact transcriptional system being evaluated. The transcriptional potentiation by nucleosome formation would appear to result from the increased specificity of the steroid hormone:receptor complex to its target organized into nucleosomes in the MMTV LTR; and once this interaction takes place, this precisely positioned nucleosome is disrupted such that the transcriptional factor NF1 now has access to its underlying specific sequence. It is of interest that the vitellogenin gene which is also potentiated by nucleosome formation is a steroid hormone responsive gene; and that other steroid hormone responsive genes are rendered non-responsive by treatment with sodium butyrate.[635] The requirement for incorporation of the steroid receptor target DNA into a precisely positioned nucleosome may be a universal feature of hormone responsive genes. Despite these few examples of augmentation of transcription as a result of nucleosome formation, in the majority of cases this organization of DNA leads to transcriptional repression. This repression can be overcome by assembly of pre-initiation complexes and sequence specific transcriptional factors in competition with histones and would argue for one level of transcriptional influence exerted by chromatin organization. While the exact influence this mechanism has on gene expression from integrated retroviruses remains to be determined, it is unlikely that these proviral sequences escape this organization.

MATRIX ATTACHMENT REGIONS (MAR/SAR)

The eukaryotic genome is organized into approximately 60,000 DNA loops with an average length of 50 kilobases (with a range of 5 to 200 kilobases) attached to a proteinaceous framework called the nuclear matrix or scaffold.[701] It is estimated that there are approximately the same number of functional genes within the eukaryotic genome. This and other data (to be discussed below) have led to the proposal that each of these DNA loops represent one gene or a small cluster of related genes with its cadre of *cis* acting regulatory sequences.[701] While the exact nature of this proteinaceous framework is poorly understood, there are two major proteins within this framework which anchor these loops at their boundaries, namely Sc1 and Sc2. Of particular note to this discussion is the recent identification of Sc1 as topoisomerase II[701] (discussed below). A number of recent reports demonstrate the influence of these matrix attachment regions on transcription.[702,708]

One of the earliest indications that integration site might influence gene expression came from construction of transgenic mice. It was noted by a number of investigators that the ultimate expression of a particular gene introduced into the fertilized mouse egg was very unpredictable; and that often there was loss of tissue and developmental regulation of this expression.[709-711] Other insight came from the elegant and in depth study of the regulation of the globin genes. It was demonstrated that this cluster of structural genes were contained within a large functional domain or chromatin loop bounded by nuclear matrix attachment regions;[712] and that the appropriate tissue and developmental expression of these genes was controlled by a number of nucleosome free hypersensitivity sites located far upstream (~20 kilobases) called the locus control region.[713-718] While not nearly as well defined as for the globin genes, it is of note that the CD4 receptor (which is a common receptor for many of the retroviruses considered herein) also requires at least 17 kilobases of upstream sequences for its tissue and appropriate developmental expression in transgenic mice.[719] Similarly, McKnight et al have shown in transgenic mice that the specific inclusion of MAR sequences flanking the whey acidic protein (WAP) transgene results in 100% expression of WAP in mammary tissue compared with only 50% expression of the transgene not containing such sequences. In addition, in four of five lines evaluated showed that there was appropriate hormonal and developmental expression of this gene.[705]

Steif et al created plasmids that either contained the basic chicken lysozyme enhancer and promoter attached to the CAT reporter gene or a similar construct with the 5' chicken lysozyme matrix attachment region (MAR) attached at both the 5' and 3' ends of this unit. There was no significant difference in expression of the CAT gene in *transient* transfections where integration did not take place. However, in cells containing stably integrated constructs, there was a dramatic increase in CAT production when the constructs contained the matrix attachment regions in the flanking position.[708] If these MAR elements were placed between the promoter/enhancer and the structural gene, however, there was complete loss of expression. This observation with the chicken lysozyme matrix attachment region has been extended to heterologous promoters and enhancers and to heterologous cell systems.[706] These relationships are illustrated schematically in Figure 3.18. There are now multiple reports of genes that have matrix attachment regions as critical components to their appropriate expression including human β interferon, human and avian β–globin, human apolipoprotein B, mouse K chain immunoglobulin, mouse whey acidic protein, rat α-macroglobulin, chicken lysozyme and several *Drosophila melanogaster* genes.[702-708] If one reasonably assumes that introduction of a randomly integrated proviral sequence into a preexisting functional domain occurs, then it too should fall under the influence of upstream (and downstream) elements which control expression of that particular chromatin loop.

In addition to the normal influence upon transcription from these MAR sequences, there is recent evidence with a number of different promoters and enhancers, including that of HIV-1, that the sodium butyrate response is mediated through these scaffold attachment sites.[704] Klehr et al have recently reported five different promoter/enhancer combinations with two reporter genes and have shown a dramatic dependence upon these sequences for maximal butyrate response.[704] It has additionally been shown with the human β interferon gene (moving upstream from the 5' end), that there is a DNase I hypersensitive site followed by a nucleosome (which is lost upon induction of transcription or treatment with butyrate) and then an extended nucleosome free region corresponding to the matrix attachment site.[702] DNA sequence analysis of these matrix attachment regions from the various genes described reveal very A-T rich stretches and usually with a topoisomerase II cleavage site within a short distance. It should be noted parenthetically that A-T rich regions are relatively resistant to nucleosome assembly even in the absence of competing nuclear matrix proteins.

Finally, viruses have been described which organize their genome via matrix attachment regions and whose replication and transcriptional properties are controlled in part by these regions, namely Epstein Barr virus[718] and Adenovirus.[719]

TOPOISOMERASE ACTIVITY

Localized torsional stresses within DNA are implicated as prerequisites (positive strain) of initiation of transcription as well as a consequence (negative strain) of the transcriptional process itself.[722] Topoisomerases are high copy number enzymes[723] associated with the nuclear matrix which mediate the cleavage/religation of either one (topoisomerase I) or both strands of DNA (topoisomerase II) which modify these torsional strains.[723,724] Topoisomerases are inhibited by a number of agents which have applications as anti-tumor agents or antimicrobial agents. Topoisomerase I is specifically inhibited by camptothecin, whereas topoisomerase II is inhibited by such agents as novobiocin, VM-26, VP-16, suramin, amsacrine, amonafide, and coumermycin A1. The mechanism of action of many of these agents is through stabilization of the covalent link between the topoisomerase and the nicked DNA at consensus sequences recognized by these enzymes, thereby preventing religation. These "cleavable complexes" in the presence of protein denaturants such as SDS or LDS produce either single strand (topoisomerase I) or double strand (topoisomerase II) breaks in DNA with the relevant topoisomerase covalently attached.[723] These cleavage sites can consequently be mapped within a given actively transcribed gene. Topoisomerase I cleavage sites have been determined for a number of genes including the human c-*fos* gene, the rat tyrosine aminotransferase gene, SV40 virus and the heat shock genes of *Drosophila*.[724,725] Similarly, sites for topoisomerase II activity have been defined for the heat shock proteins of Drosophila, the human c-*myc* gene, chicken B-globin genes and SV40 genome in infected monkey cells.[724] As might be expected, the topoisomerase II cleavage sites were clustered at matrix attachment sites flanking both the 5' and 3' ends of genes. In addition to the agents that act at the step of religation, there are several of these agents whose mechanism of action is prevention of the initial cleavage event.

It is of note that suramin has recently been shown to be a potent inhibitor of topoisomerase II.[726] Suramin was shown earlier in tissue culture to reduce HIV-1 viral replication which was assumed to be due to reverse transcriptase activity.[727,728] It was also successful in reducing circulating viral levels in a small number of patients,[729,730] however, due to toxicity and variability of response, it has not been adopted as standard care for HIV-1 infected patients.[731,732] Laughlin et al showed that another topoisomerase II inhibitor, novobiocin, has similar effects on induction of viral replication in a chronically infected, nonpermissive CD4 negative cell line. We demonstrated that the synergistic effect of sodium butyrate and phorbol esters could be blocked in the presence of novobiocin.[700]

CONCLUSION

It is our hypothesis that there are multiple levels of transcriptional regulation which a cell can bring to bear on either native cellular genes or integrated proviral genes. One such level of regulation is inducible sequence-specific transcriptional factors which have been extensively investigated with respect to the HIV-1 LTR. This level of control can be modified by organization of the DNA into nucleosomes either by directly excluding these sequence specific transcriptional factors or by modifying the torsional stresses within the target DNA; and further modified by higher order chromatin structures bounded by nuclear matrix attachment sequences. Transcription from within these chromatin loops or domains may be limited (or propagated) by torsional stresses on local stretches of DNA under the influence of topoisomerase II activity located within the nuclear matrix at these attachment sites. It might be predicted then that the level of viral replication in the clinical setting is determined to a large extent by the relatively ran-

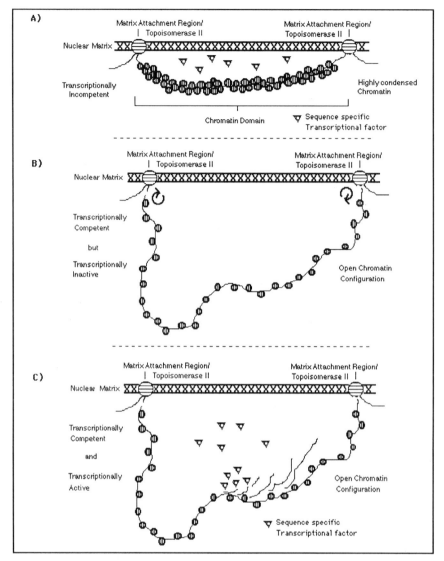

Fig. 3.18. Hypothetical model of transcriptional regulation by chromatin structure. Gene clusters are organized into chromatin domains whose 5' and 3' ends are anchored to the proteinacous nuclear matrix. Matrix attachment regions (MARs) are short 100-400 base pair sequences (with a very high A + T content) which are bound to topoisomerase II enzymes incorporated within the nuclear matrix. The attachment of the double stranded DNA to the nuclear matrix impedes its rotational freedom and can thereby maintain a particular chromatin domain (i.e., gene cluster) in either an open or closed configuration in isolation from neighboring chromatin domains. As shown in panel A, chromatin maintained in a highly condensed configuration is inactive (transcriptionally incompetent) presumably due to lack of access to transcriptional factors and perhaps lack of rotational freedom. In panel B, there is an unspecified signal which results in the double stranded cleavage of DNA by topoisomerase II at the MAR site with "unraveling" of the chromatin fiber into an open configuration with subsequent religation of DNA by topoisomerase II. This chromatin re-organization now generates a transcriptionally competent chromatin configuration; but remains inactive in the absence of induction of sequence specific transcriptional factors. In panel C, there is transcriptional activation as a result of induction of sequence specific transcriptional factors which can now find their target and assemble the transcriptional protein complex.

dom integration event of HIV-1 and the mitigating influence of surrounding genomic DNA. Beyond this cellularly determined regulation of HIV-1 gene expression, there are the viral gene products themselves that participate in the rate of transcriptional initiation and more importantly, in the efficiency of transcriptional elongation (*tat*) and the ultimate fate of those initiated transcripts (*rev*). The apparent high number of non-productively infected mononuclear cells present early in clinical infection may reflect a selection pressure for integrative events leading to latent infection by a healthy immune system which clears those cells actively producing virus. As the immune system fails either by slow CD4 depletion or amplification of escape mutants of the virus, there is a progressive increase in cells actively replicating HIV-1 which in turn leads to further potential for integration into transcriptionally active regions of the genome.

A clinical strategy resulting from such a proposal would be to shift the majority of anti-retroviral therapy to the earliest stages of HIV-1 infection with the intent to prevent subsequent rounds of infection which have the potential to integrate into active chromatin; or which would provide the potential substrate for generation of escape mutants. In addition, therapy aimed at prevention of chromatin structural alterations (which results from PBMC activation in response to circulating cytokines or antigen specific stimulation) might prove to be another approach to HIV-1 treatment in conjunction with anti-retroviral therapy. Two potentially promising future points of intervention in this regard are topoisomerase II inhibitors which might have value during periods of intercurrent infections to dampen chromatin re-organization; and agents which block the effects of circulating cytokines such as thalidimide which is currently under clinical investigation as an anti-TNF-α. While much remains to be established the ultimate successful management of HIV-1 infection will likely require intervention at each of the multiple levels of HIV-1 transcriptional control.

===================== CHAPTER 4 =====================

OTHER HUMAN AND NON-HUMAN PRIMATE RETROVIRUSES

As discussed in detail in chapters 2 and 3, there are a multitude of determinants of retroviral gene expression. From the moment of integration of the retroviral sequences into the host's genome, there are an array of viral and cellular factors that contribute to the ultimate level of retroviral replication. In addition, the unique life cycle of retroviruses which results in the placement of their proviral sequence within the context of cellular chromatin subjects them to further transcriptional regulation. Given the complexity of these many transcriptional regulatory pathways, another approach to deciphering the pathogenesis of retroviral infections is by comparison of the replicative ability of many different (but related) retroviruses within their respective hosts. As discussed in chapter 1, there are markedly different biological behaviors among the many human and non-human primate retroviruses studied. HIV-1 and its closely related simian counterpart SIVcpz share a great deal of sequence homology and yet have quite different "disease penetrance" in their respective hosts. Similarly, SIVsm/mac infection of sooty mangabeys leads to no apparent disease while SIVsm/mac infection of rhesus macaques results in an immunodeficiency syndrome reminiscent of AIDS. HIV-2 which is closely related to this SIVsm/mac results in an immunodeficiency syndrome in humans but with significantly different kinetics from HIV-1. The human T-cell lymphoma/leukemia viruses I and II are closely related structurally and yet they have dramatically different clinical outcomes. Acquisition of HTLV-I in infancy leads in a minority of cases to adult T-cell leukemia in southern Japan; yet leads to a myelopathic syndrome when acquired later in life in the Caribbean Basin. HTLV-II which can be found in isolated pockets throughout the world has no apparent "disease penetrance." Similar to HTLV-II, the Spumaviruses are not convincingly associated, as yet, with any human or simian disease. We will examine a select few of these retroviral:host interactions and review the available data on their transcriptional control in direct comparison to what is known of these mechanisms for HIV-1.

HUMAN IMMUNODEFICIENCY VIRUS TYPE 2 (HIV-2)

There is mounting evidence that the clinical course leading to immunodeficiency with HIV-2 is slower than with HIV-1.[35,733-738] HIV-2 was first identified from West Africa and, unlike HIV-1 which has rapidly spread throughout the world, HIV-2 has remained largely confined geographically.[35] In addition, serological data would suggest that HIV-2 was present within this population prior to the arrival of HIV-1, perhaps as early as the 1960s.[739,740] Other epidemiological data also support a lower "virulence" with HIV-2. The rate of perinatal transmission with HIV-2 is significantly less than with HIV-1;[741,742] and there is a different age-specific prevalence of infection between these two pathogens.[743-746] In one study, the highest prevalence rate for HIV-1 infection in women was in the under-20 age group. In contrast, for infection with HIV-2 the highest prevalence rate was from age 30-39. In addition, the ratio of HIV-1 infection to HIV-2 infection within this same population showed a decreasing prevalence ratio; that is, in the under-20 age group there was a 16.8 to 1 ratio of HIV-1 to HIV-2 infection. Within the over 40 age group, however, the ratio had fallen to 2.5 to 1.[35] There are a number of possibilities to account for these findings. One potential reason for the declining ratio might be that the incidence of acquisition of HIV-2 increases with age (i.e. highest prevalence is in the older groups) which will increase the denominator (HIV-2 infection); in addition, there may be a selective loss of HIV-1 infected people to death which will decrease the numerator (HIV-1 infection) with the combined effect of reducing the prevalence ratios. Alternatively, although the routes of transmission between these two pathogens appears to be identical, transmissibility between HIV-1 and HIV-2 might differ resulting in a greater number of people acquiring HIV-1 sooner; but with continued exposures more people become infected with HIV-2 and the prevalence of those infected with HIV-2 "catches up" with HIV-1. While there are certainly other possibilities, there is at least some preliminary evidence to support this latter proposal. Serological data from prostitutes in Abidjan, Ivory Coast show a greater than 40% prevalence of HIV-2 infection among those already infected with HIV-1.[35] By contrast, there is a less than 5% prevalence of seropositivity for HIV-2 alone.[35] This would suggest that risk behaviors for acquisition of infection results in acquisition of HIV-1 more often than HIV-2; but with continued exposure there is accumulation of HIV-2 seroreactivity. Similarly, a survey of seroconversion among blood donors from Ivory Coast in 1991 identified a 27:1 ratio of seroconversion to HIV-1 compared with HIV-2.[747] The ratio of HIV-1 to HIV-2 seroprevalence among this same donor population however, was only 6:1 arguing against the trivial explanation that these differences in age-specific prevalence merely reflect the respective rates of infection with HIV-1 and HIV-2 within the population.[747]

The recent study by Marlink et al further substantiates the divergent clinical progression between HIV-1 and HIV-2 infection.[738] These investigators identified a cohort of HIV-1 and HIV-2 seropositive women whom they followed for 7-8 years. Among those identified as seroconverter (i.e. time zero of infection), there was a 100% disease free survival at 5 years in the HIV-2 infected women; by comparison, the HIV-1 infected women had only a 67% five year disease survival. In addition to having a greater likelihood of remaining disease free, the HIV-2 group also had a significantly greater likelihood of maintaining a normal CD4+ T-lymphocyte count.

Finally, initial attempts to quantitate and compare viral burden/viremia between HIV-1 and HIV-2 show a significantly lower level of viral detection in HIV-2 infected people, at least in the asymptomatic stages of infection.[35,748,] Simon et al showed that with CD4+ T-cell counts over 500, they could isolate virus in 92% of HIV-1 infected people while they isolated virus in only 18% of those infected with HIV-2.[748] Similarly with CD4+ counts between 200 and 500, virus was isolated in 94% of HIV-1 infected people and in 62% of HIV-2 infected people. By the time of clinical immunosuppression (i.e., CD4+ cell counts below 200), however, they could isolate virus from 100% of HIV-1 and HIV-2 infected people.[748] This would suggest that there may be less viral replication during early infection with HIV-2 than with HIV-1. This might also account for the lower perinatal transmission rate. While the mechanism of perinatal transmission is unknown, there is some evidence to suggest that the level of viremia is associated with the incidence of transmission.[749] If, in fact, there is a lower viremia in HIV-2 infection prior to immunosuppression (and immunosuppression occurs later than in HIV-1), then it might be expected that the incidence of perinatal transmission would be different between the two viruses. It is tempting to draw the simple conclusion that the apparent slower replication rate with HIV-2 is directly responsible for the slower clinical progression. Considered within the context of the hypothetical model of HIV pathogenesis presented in Figure 2.13A (chapter 2), a slower rate of replication would lead to less immune destruction of CD4+ cells and to fewer opportunities for mutant virus generation by the low fidelity reverse transcriptase enzyme. This would statistically predict an increase in the time required to move from Phase III to Phase IV.

If we assume that there is in fact a difference in the level of viral gene expression between HIV-1 and HIV-2, then a closer look at the HIV-2 viral regulatory elements is required. As discussed for HIV-1, the four major areas to scrutinize in terms of transcriptional control are the regulatory proteins (i) *tat* and (ii) *rev*, the (iii) LTR and (iv) the impact of surrounding chromatin structures on these elements. Since there is essentially no specific data available on chromatin structure and HIV-2 we will concentrate on the first three of these regulatory elements.

The full length HIV-2 *tat* protein is 130 amino acids in comparison to 86 for HIV-1 *tat*. Like HIV-1 *tat*, HIV-2 *tat* is derived from two exons and contains a cysteine rich region, a transactivation domain, and an arginine rich TAR RNA binding region; and like HIV-1 *tat* there are reports of full functional activity of the single exon (99 amino acid) of HIV-2 *tat* protein.[750-756] Beyond these conserved regions, however, there is little sequence homology between the two *tat* proteins. Mutational analyses have identified a number of features which distinguish HIV-2 *tat* from HIV-1 *tat*. Arya reports that approximately 20% of the amino terminal portion of the HIV-2 *tat* molecule can be deleted without loss of function; and approximately 30% of the carboxy terminal portion is dispensable for function.[754] Echetebu and Rice similarly demonstrate that the carboxy terminal region from approximately amino acid 90 and up can be deleted with maintenance of function.[752] They also identified a critical region within the amino terminal region (from amino acid 8 through 47) which is critical to transactivation function. These results are somewhat contradictory to Arya's laboratory mutational analyses which report that amino acids 12-37 are non-essential; that loss of amino acids 1 through 10 reduce transactivation somewhat; and that residues 38-47 are essential.[754] Echetebu and Rice find that loss of amino acids 8 through 33 markedly reduce transactivating potential while loss of amino acid residues 8 through 47 abolish *tat* function.[752] One possible reconciliation of these data would be the critical requirement of amino acids in positions 8-10 which accounts for the lowered function in Arya's 1-10 deletion and Echetebu and Rice's 8-33 deletion, with residues 11-33 being non-contributory to this loss of function. The evidence from both laboratories are compatible with the essential nature of residues 38-47. Echetebu and Rice provide further evidence of the unique nature of each viral *tat* protein by constructing chimeric proteins between HIV-1 and HIV-2.[752] They made reciprocal exchanges of the amino terminal portions of both *tat* proteins up to the first cysteine residue; that is, they placed the amino terminal portion of HIV-1 *tat* in the position of the amino terminal portion of HIV-2 *tat* and the amino terminal portion of HIV-2 *tat* in the position of HIV-1 *tat*. Each of these chimerics would be expected to recognize and bind its target site on their respective TAR RNAs; however, there was loss of function for each.[752] These data would suggest that each tat's transactivating mechanism(s) (or requirements) is different. Finally, one of the HIV-2 *tat* mutants created by Echetebu and Rice which deletes within the basic domain (TAR RNA binding function and nuclear localizing function) resulted in a transdominant negative inhibitor of both HIV-1 and HIV-2.[753] This would suggest that the *tat* "co-factor" as discussed in chapter 2 may be shared between the two *tat* proteins.

Finally, it is widely reported that the HIV-1 *tat* protein can fully transactivate both the HIV-1 LTR as well as the HIV-2 LTR; whereas the HIV-2 *tat* protein can only fully transactivate the HIV-2 LTR.[750,756-758] A recent report has, however, questioned this conclusion. Tong-Starksen et al have provided evidence that the HIV-2 *tat* protein can indeed transactivate the HIV-1 LTR if both exons are present (which requires expression from plasmids with cDNA of full length *tat* and not with genomic constructs).[759] Another obvious difference between HIV-1 and HIV-2 *tat* transactivational function is the target TAR RNA. While the HIV-1 TAR element is contained within nucleotides +14 to +45, that of HIV-2 extends from +1 to +90.[750,758] In addition, the HIV-2 TAR RNA contains tandem stem-loop structures rather than a single stem loop as for HIV-1. Like the HIV-1 TAR RNA however, the HIV-2 TAR RNA secondary structure contains a small bulge (dinucleotide in the case if HIV-2 and trinucleotide in the case of HIV-1) in the ascending limb of the stem; and the loop structures are necessary for full transactivational potential.[750,758,760] The predicted TAR RNA secondary structure is shown in Figure 4.19. Mutational analysis of this region has demonstrated that each stem-loop structure can function independently of the other but that the 5' stem-loop is more functionally significant.[758,761] To complete the analogy with the HIV-1 TAR stem-loop structure, Rhim and Rice investigated the function of the dinucleotide bulges within each of these two stem-loops.[760] They found that deletion of both dinucleotide bulges eliminated *tat* binding and *tat* transactivation. Deletion of only the 5' bulge reduced *tat* function (~30% of wild type) but binding was maintained as demonstrated by in vitro nuclease protection assays. In contrast, deletion of only the 3' dinucleotide bulge had no impact on *tat*'s transactivating ability nor on TAR RNA binding.[760]

In summary, HIV-1 and HIV-2 *tat* proteins are significantly divergent on a sequence basis but share critical functional domains; both proteins transactivate by increasing the steady state level of their respective proviral specific mRNAs; both are derived from two exons but with the second exon of questionable functional significance (at least in vitro); and both appear to interact with a (perhaps the same) cellular co-factor. The "host range" for HIV-1 *tat* appears somewhat

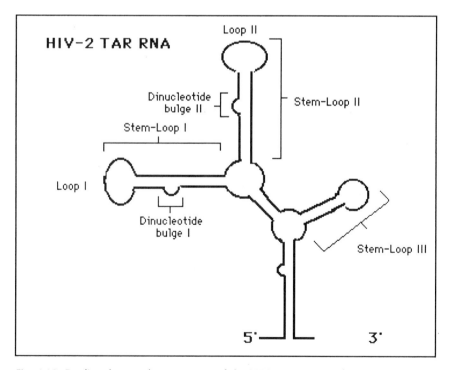

Fig. 4.19. Predicted secondary structure of the HIV-2 TAR RNA. The HIV-2 TAR RNA secondary structure contains tandem stem-loop structures and as such is significantly larger than the HIV-1 TAR region. Like HIV-1, the HIV-2 TAR RNA has a small bulge in the ascending limb of its stem implicated in tat binding; and the loop structures are required for full activity.

larger than for HIV-2 in that HIV-1 *tat* fully transactivates both the HIV-1 LTR and HIV-2 LTR; whereas the HIV-2 *tat* protein is most efficient at transactivating its own LTR. Finally, the HIV-2 TAR RNA target contains two functional stem-loop structures in tandem, each with a dinucleotide bulge and each with an essential loop sequence for the presumptive binding of a cellular protein.

A comparison of the *rev* proteins between HIV-1 and HIV-2 show a similar pattern of shared and non-shared features. The *rev* protein of HIV-2 is similar to HIV-1 in its functional domain composition in that it has the basic nuclear localizing domain which also functions as the RNA binding domain; the leucine rich activation domain; and multimerization regions.[761-764] In contrast, however, the HIV-2 *rev* response element (RRE) has a markedly different primary sequence as well as a significantly different predicted secondary structure as shown in Figure 4.20. Furthermore, *rev* from HIV-1 can efficiently transactivate both the HIV-1 RRE and the HIV-2 RRE. In contrast, the HIV-2 *rev* protein can only transactivate its own RRE.[761-764] Whether the differences in *tat* and *rev* structure and function between these two retroviruses can account for the apparent differences in the replicative rates of HIV-1 and HIV-2 in vivo remains uncertain.

The LTRs from HIV-2 isolates (as well as from SIV isolates—see below) are somewhat longer than for HIV-1 isolates. Most HIV-1 LTRs

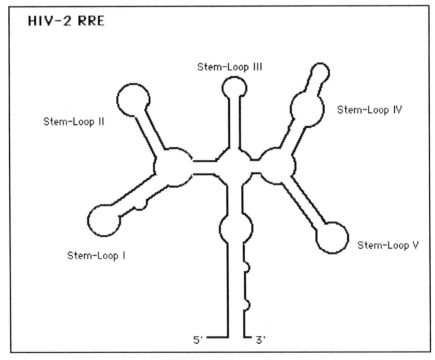

Fig. 4.20. HIV-2 Rev Response Element (RRE). The predicted secondary structure of the HIV-2 RRE. While significantly different from the HIV-1 RRE, the HIV-1 rev protein can recognize the HIV-2 RRE and transactivate it; whereas, the HIV-2 rev protein can only transactivate the HIV-2 RRE and not that of HIV-1.

are approximately 630 base pairs in length while LTRs of HIV-2 are closer to 800 base pairs in length. Some of this difference in LTR length is contributed by the larger TAR region in HIV-2. In addition, HIV-2 (and SIVsm/mac) isolates contain four potential Sp-1 binding sites compared with the three for HIV-1.[765] As in the HIV-1 LTR, upstream of the Sp-1 sites in the HIV-2 LTR lies an NF-κB binding site; however, the HIV-2 LTR only contains one functional NF-κB site rather than the two found in HIV-1.[766-769] Although the HIV-2 LTR has received much less investigation than the exhaustively probed HIV-1 LTR, Markovitz et al demonstrated four critical regulatory sequences within the HIV-2 LTR.[768] Two of these sites are designated PuB1 and PuB2. PuB1 lies from -174 to -160 and PuB2 lies between -142 and -135. These purine rich regions bind members of the ETS family of transcriptional factors. Between these two ETS binding sites (-153 to -144) lies another critical element, the peri-ETS or pets, site. The fourth critical regulatory sequence is the single NF-κB site.[768-770] In a direct comparison between HIV-1 and HIV-2 transcriptional response, Hilfinger et al report that in a monocytic cell line, the HIV-2 response to phorbol ester stimulation is dependent upon all four sites; whereas with HIV-1, the majority of response to either phorbol ester stimulation or developmentally regulated viral expression are mediated through the two NF-κB sites.[769] A similar differential regulation between HIV-1 and HIV-2 was demonstrated by Hannibal et al in response to physiological T-cell activation signals.[770] They found that HIV-2 was poorly responsive to either stimulation with TNF-α or to over-expression of the cloned NF-κB subunits, both of which potently stimulate HIV-1 expression. By contrast, T-cell receptor (TCR):CD3 signaling was very efficient in transactivating the HIV-2 LTR.[770]

While much less is known of the HIV-2 LTR, the principles of transcriptional regulation as outlined for HIV-1 are likely to participate in its level of expression. As discussed, there are some differences between the HIV-1 and HIV-2 LTRs and their overall sequence homology is only approximately 45%; however, the functional organization of the core enhancer and promoter share many features between the viruses. Both contain a TATA box with Sp-1 sites immediately upstream. Both have NF-κB sites upstream of the Sp-1 sites, although HIV-2 contains only one. As will be discussed below, one of the mutations found in the highly virulent variant of SIVsm (when compared with the parent virus) was a duplicated NF-κB site. On the other hand, virulence failed to map strictly to this site and some SIVs have no recognizable NF-κB sites and yet effectively replicate within their hosts.[765] Both HIV-1 and HIV-2 have TAR DNA elements which generate highly structured RNAs that serve as targets for *tat*'s transactivation. Whether the apparently greater promiscuity of HIV-1 *tat* for heterologous TAR elements participates in the generation of higher plasma viremia in HIV-1 infection compared with HIV-2 infection remains to be determined. A similar question could be framed for the *rev* and *rev*:RRE difference between viruses. As with *tat*, the HIV-1 *rev* protein is somewhat more promiscuous in its target selection than HIV-2's *rev*. As with the theme of "incrementalism" developed for transcriptional control of HIV-1, the ultimate level of HIV-2 gene expression will likely be the result of all of these (and probably more) subtle differences. Furthermore, one could speculate that with a lower baseline level of viral replication early in infection, there are fewer opportunities for integration into transcriptionally active chromatin domains leading to fewer cells which replicate virus that subsequently become targets for immune destruction and less of a taxation of the CD4+ lymphocyte population.

SIMIAN IMMUNODEFICIENCY VIRUS(ES)

The simian immunodeficiency viruses (SIVs) are a diverse group of retroviruses consisting of five major subgroups: (i) SIVagm, (ii) SIVcpz, (iii) SIVsyk; (iv) SIVmnd; and (v) SIVsm/mac.[1,771] While their study will no doubt yield a greater understanding of the pathogenesis of their human counterparts, HIV-1 and HIV-2, many representatives of these subgroups have yet to be investigated in detail. In addition, there has proven to be a remarkably variable "disease penetrance" among these agents depending upon which strains (and substrains) are studied and in which host; and depending upon the cell culture passage history of the virus.[771] Attempts to categorize these many retroviruses in terms of their relative pathogenicity have failed to yield a clear identification of a virally determined pathogenic moiety. In terms of this discussion, we will briefly examine only three groups: (i) SIVagm, (ii) SIVcpz, and (iii) SIVsm/mac.

SIVagm

Nearly 50% of African green monkeys are infected with this retrovirus in the wild and yet there is no apparent disease in its native host.[1,2] Its study in other species has been limited primarily by its lack of pathogenicity. A number of investigators have attempted infection of macaques with SIVagm.[772-775] Gravell et al were able to induce a fatal immunodefieicncy in one pigtail macaque with strain 155 of SIVagm; however, further attempts to induce disease in either rhesus or pigtail macaques failed.[771,773,774] Another strain, SIVagm90, did cause immunodeficiency in two pigtail macaques, one fatal and the other with a persistently low CD4 lymphocyte count.[774] Given its relatively low virulence in cross-species infections and its total lack of pathogenicity in it native host, SIVagm has received relatively little study. One laboratory did attempt to quantitate viral load in naturally infected African green monkeys.[776] Hartung et al examined viral DNA burden by end point dilution DNA PCR and found a mean of 15 copies of SIVagm specific proviral sequences per 10^5 peripheral blood mononuclear cells (PBMCs). In addition, by end point dilution culturing of PBMCs from 17 seropositive animals, they could recover virus in 14 of the 17; and in those animal from which they did recover virus, approximately 1 in 10^5 cells carried "rescueable" SIVagm. Finally, only 4 of the 17 animals had detectable plasma viremia (similar to HIV-2 infected people with high CD4 lymphocyte count[748]).[776] Comparison of these limited data with levels of viral burden in early, asymptomatic HIV-1 and HIV-2 infection show some similarity. Hirsch and Johnson extended these findings by comparing viral burden between SIVagm infected African green monkeys and SIVsm infected macaques.[771] They also found comparable viral burdens between these two animal groups while the macaques were healthy. As the macaques developed symptomatic disease, however, there was a dramatic increase in tissue and plasma viral load (just as there is in humans).[771] While these data confirm the observations with HIV-1 and HIV-2, that the level of viral replication within the host is correlated with clinical disease progression, these studies do not shed any light on the mechanisms by which naturally infected African green monkeys limit their viral replication throughout their lifetime. In an attempt to define the role of the LTR in SIVagm gene expression, Sakuragi et al linked a number of different SIV and HIV LTRs to a reporter gene and assayed their function.[777] They found that the LTRs from four different strains of SIVagm were actually much more active at baseline than were LTRs derived from HIV-1, HIV-2, SIVsm or SIVmnd. In the presence of *tat*, however, the other LTRs showed greater relative transactivation.[777] These findings are consistent with the data from *tat* transactivation of the HIV-1 LTR; that is, under conditions where there is high processivity of transcripts at baseline, there is relatively less transactivation by *tat*, whereas under conditions of low processivity *tat*'s effects are more prominent. What is surprising about these findings, however, is the relatively greater baseline activity of the SIVagm LTRs which would not be expected in light of lower levels of viral replication in vivo. It is obvious from these data that in vitro studies using transient transfection assays need cautious interpretation; and that much more investigation is required to determine the precise host:virus interaction in African green monkeys which maintains lifelong transcriptional control over their proviral sequences.

SIVcpz

As discussed elsewhere, SIVcpz is very closely related to HIV-1 and may have been its origin within the human population. As a result, many of its structural elements are very similar to those of HIV-1. What is not similar, however, is its apparent total lack of disease potential in chimpanzees despite the clear establishment of infection.[13-22] There have been more than 100 chimpanzees inoculated with human isolates and to date none have developed AIDS.[778] Attempts to define viral load in chimpanzees have yielded similar results to those of African green monkeys discussed above. Saksela et al determined that in infected chimpanzees, there are approximately 1 in 10^4 to 1 in 10^5 PBMC which harbor HIV-1 proviral DNA and markedly fewer which spontaneously express HIV-1 specific mRNA. Of note, was the ease of induction of mRNA in vitro from many of these latently infected PBMC suggesting that these proviral sequences are intact. Also, reminiscent of human infection, there was a higher viral burden within lymphatic tissue of these infected animals.

It should be noted that we are assuming a significantly high enough homology between HIV-1 and SIVcpz to discuss SIVcpz in terms of chimpanzees infected with human isolates of HIV-1. While this assumption may not be entirely justified, there are no data available on primate infection with SIVcpz isolates from feral chimpanzees. While few conclusions can be drawn with the limited data available, these observations would reinforce the concept that the disease potential of HIV-1 lies not in its precise sequence but rather in the host:virus interaction.

SIVsm/mac

SIVsm/mac is the most widely studied of the simian immunodeficiency viruses. One reason for the great interest in this subgroup of viruses is its similar pathogenic potential to HIV-1. It was first isolated around the time of the initial clinical descriptions of AIDS. There was an "outbreak" of immunodeficiency associated illness and of lymphomas within a colony of macaques at the New England Regional Primate Research Center in the early 1980s.[779-781] It was soon demonstrated that this immunodeficiency syndrome could be passaged by inoculation of tissue filtrates into other macaques.[782,783] Isolation of a very homologous virus from sooty mangabeys (SIVsm) and from West African patients (HIV-2) with AIDS further defined this valuable animal model of AIDS. Many of the clinical features of immunodeficiency induced by SIVsm/mac infection of macaques are similar to human infection with either HIV-1 or HIV-2. In many animals there is progressive loss of CD4+ lymphocytes with ultimate development of opportunistic infections, development of a wasting syndrome and clinically apparent involvement of the central nervous system.[24] Similarly, the immunological events surrounding the initial infection and control of the acute viremia are comparable; that is, there is generation of SIV specific cytotoxic T-cells in addition to antibody production which effectively reduces the initial plasma viremia.[784] There seems to be one of three outcomes that follow this initial course of events in SIVsm/mac infected macaques: (i) relatively rapid progression to immunodeficiency and death, usually in the absence of an effective immune response; (ii) development of low grade persistent viremia lasting 1 to 3 years with the subsequent development of simian AIDS; and in a small number of animals (iii) loss of detectable viremia in the face of a persistent immune response.[24] In this latter circumstance, there is ready detection of proviral sequences by PCR of PBMCs but rare isolation of virus. The ultimate outcome for these animals is uncertain but some have lived for years.[24] It is of interest that there are a handfull of reports of humans who also maintain an HIV-1 specific immune reactivity without detectable viremia after many years and the prediction that there will be a small minority of HIV-1 infected people who never develop disease (personal communication to Pomerantz).[785] Within the hypothetical model of HIV-1 pathogenesis presented in Figs. 2.13A, B) one could speculate that in rare cases, the initial clearing of productively infected cells by HIV-1 specific CTLs leaves no cells which have integrated provirus into chromatin regions which are capable of re-activation; or that the very few cells which do contain provirus within chromatin region which have the potential to reactivate do not do so because they never encounter the necessary antigen specific signal.

At the other end of the clinical spectrum of SIVsm/mac infection is the extensively investigated rapidly fatal variant of SIVsm termed SIVsmmPBj14. This viral isolate originated from a pig-tailed macaque infected with SIVsmm9. This animal (serial number PBj) died at 14 months post-infection with an AIDS-like illness and its whole blood was injected into several recipient animals who subsequently developed acute illness. Two of these animals died within days and another within a few weeks of inoculation.[29,786] Molecular clones from viral isolates of these animals were derived and several such clones proved to establish rapidly progressive (and fatal) disease identical to the original biological clone in a variety of species.[786-789] Of particular interest, the original parental isolate was from a sooty mangabey in which there was no disease production; however, after passage through pig-tailed macaques and molecular cloning, the SIV-PBj14 variant became pathogenic in sooty mangabeys.[790] Sequence analysis of these two viruses, SIVsmm9 and its derivative SIV-PBj14, by Courgnaud et al identified a number of significant features. They suggest that a maximum of 57 point mutations within the SIVsmm9 provirus plus a 22 base pair insertion into the LTR and a 15 base pair insertion into the env gene could account for the newly acquired lethal nature of SIV-PBj14. It is of note that the LTR insertion is of an NF-κB like enhancer. They further suggest that there is a positive immune selective pressure for the 5 amino acid change resulting from the env insertion. Attempts to generate chimeric proviruses between lethal and non-lethal molecular clones suggested multiple determinants were responsible for this newly acquired virulence.[791] Novembre et al showed that the new env gene was required for this virulence but that it required other elements of the virulent strain as well. Of note, they did not find that the duplicated NF-κB element was required for this new phenotype.[791] Within the context of the discussion of the pathogenesis of HIV-1, it may be that the significant difference between this virulent strain and its non-virulent counterpart lies predominantly within Phase I disease as depicted in Figure 2.13B. Within the model presented, it is suggested that acute HIV-1 infection is similar to most other acute viral infections in that there is early unchecked viral replication; and what sets it apart is the persistence of integrated proviral sequences after the immune destruction of cells actively expressing viruses with the consequent establishment of chronic infection. If in the case of SIV-PBj14, because of the env mutation, there is an inability to mount this initial immune response, then there is no progression to Phase II and the animal dies of an uncontrolled acute viral syndrome. In support of such a model, there are reports of a few animals who survive the initial acute viral stages of SIV-PBj14 who then go on to establishment of the prototypic chronic infection.[788] The exact contribution of the other "helper" genes derived from the virulent strain remain unknown. It might be predicted that if any of these other mutated genes lead to increased transcriptional activity (in addition to retardation of the immune response contributed by the env mutation), there would be a greater likelihood of overwhelming infection.

There have been other attempts to clearly define a virulence moiety within strains of SIVsm/mac. Marthas et al made chimeric viruses derived from the pathogenic strain SIVmac239 and the non-pathogenic strain SIVmac1A11.[792-794] They took an internal 6.2 kilobase fragment from one virus and placed it in the context of the other virus. In addition, they made other chimerics with only a 1.4 kilobase env region exchanged between viruses. These constructs generated four chimeric viruses and two parental strains which were subsequently injected into rhesus macaques.[792] The pathogenic SIVmac239 parental strain produced AIDS in all four animals within two years of injection, with three fatalities. One animal out of four receiving the chimeric with the 5' and 3' ends derived from SIVmac239 and the internal 6.2 kilobases from SIVmac1A11 developed AIDS. Similarly, one out of four animals receiving the chimeric virus containing the 5' and 3' ends from the non-pathogenic SIVmac1A11 strain with the internal 6.2 kilobases from SIVmac239 developed AIDS. None of the other animals receiving either chimeric viruses or the parental non-pathogenic virus SIVmac1A11 developed disease. All 24 animals injected developed an acute viremia within the first 4 weeks of observation and all of the SIVmac1A11 injected animals cleared their viremia. Similar to the SIV-PBj14/SIVsmm9 analysis, these data suggest that the pathogenicity of simian immunodeficiency virus infection of macaques is multi-factorial with contributions from several regions of the proviral genome and these contributions are likely influenced by the individual host being infected. Finally, as suggested in the discussion of the HIV-2 LTR, the SIV LTRs have somewhat different transcriptional features compared with HIV-1.[765,795] In addition, given the high sequence homology between SIVsm/mac and HIV-2, much of the discussion of the HIV-2 LTR is interchangeable with the SIVsm/mac LTR. One of the distinguishing features of the SIVsm/mac LTR is the relatively less critical nature of the NF-κB sequences. Bellas et al demonstrated that mutation of the single NF-κB site in the SIVmac239 strain did not significantly alter its replication in either established CD4+ cell lines or peripheral blood lymphocytes.[796]

It is clear that the simian immunodeficiency viruses will provide a powerful model in which to bridge the large gap between the enormous body of in vitro data on HIV-1 replication and its pathogenesis in vivo. While there is far less data on each individual SIV compared with HIV-1, much of the data that is available supports the pathogenesis model presented for HIV-1. It would seem that transition from Phase I to Phase II (Fig. 2.13B) in SIV infection involves the generation of an SIV-specifc immune response; and in the absence of this immune response there follows an acutely lethal infection. If and when this transition is made, there is reduction of plasma viremia and transition into the clinically latent Phase III. It would appear to be this phase in which the host:virus interaction is established which either leads to lifelong levels of "tolerable" viral gene expression or to a slow drift toward Phase IV with CD4+ depletion, opportunistic infection, overwhelming viremia and death.

HUMAN T-CELL LEUKEMIA VIRUSES

While more distantly related to HIV-1 than the other human and simian lentiviruses, the human T-cell leukemia viruses (HTLVs) type I and II share many essential features with HIV-1 in terms of clinical latency, genomic organization and use of regulatory proteins. HIV-1 was in fact classified as a member of the HTLV family, HTLV-III, for several years following its isolation. We will not exhaustively review the large body of literature on the HTLVs but briefly examine a selected few aspects of their molecular biology as it relates to retroviral latency. It is of interest that the HTLVs, like the HIVs, have a simian counterpart. Simian T-cell leukemia virus (STLV) has been described in a number of Old World monkeys and apes[797-799] and LTR sequence analysis of HTLV-I and STLV shows high sequence homology.[800-802] An interesting recent phylogenetic analysis of a large number of HTLV and STLV viral isolates has suggested the existence of these viruses for centuries; but more significantly, examination of phylogenetic clusters of HTLVs and STLVs suggest that rather than a single interspecies transmission with independent evolution of these viruses in their respective hosts, there has been a number of ongoing interspecies transmissions throughout the evolution of both.[803] Similarly, HTLV II appears to have diverged from HTLV I/STLV prior to the divergence of HTLV I from STLV.[801]

The clinical manifestations of STLV infection in the wild parallels the adult T-cell leukemia (ATL) seen in humans; however there is no evidence to date of a simian counterpart to the neuropathic disease as seen in humans infected in the Caribbean basin.[803-806] Epidemiological studies of HTLV I have established essentially three major routes of transmission: (i) male-to-female sexual transmission (but little or no female-to-male transmission); (ii) mother-to-child transmission via breast milk; and (iii) blood transfusion.[800,807-811] While the mode of transmission of HTLV II is less well studied, recent serological and PCR data from intravenous drug users supports blood product transmission as one potential route.[812,813]

The genomic organization of HTLV-I and HTLV-II are similar to the lentiviruses discussed above. They are approximately 9.0 and 8.9 kilobases in length respectively.[814,815] Five essential gene regions are defined: (i) gag; (ii); protease; (iii) pol; (iv) env; and (v) pX.[800] As with the lentiviruses, the mRNA pattern of expression is complex. The doubly spliced mRNA from the pX gene generates three proteins: (i) *tax*/p40; (ii) *rex*/p27; and (iii) p21 whose function remains to be defined. Also like lentiviruses, the *tax* and *rex* proteins are critical to the level of viral gene expression of HTLV-I and HTLV-II. The *tax* protein is functionally similar to the HIV-1 and HIV-2 *tat* proteins in that it transactivates the HTLV LTR.[76,816,817] Unlike *tat* however, *tax* does not interact with an RNA target; nor does it directly bind DNA.[818,819] The DNA target sequence for *tax* transactivation is a series of three 21 base pair repeats within the LTR, the core of which is the pentanucleotide sequence TGACG. This sequence has been defined as the recognition site for the CREB/ATF family of transcriptional factors.[76,820-822] Since direct DNA binding has not been demonstrated, it has been widely assumed that *tax* interacts with the CREB/ATF-like factor which in turn is bound to this target sequence.[76] In addition to interaction with the CREB/ATF family of transcriptional factors, *tax* also interacts with NF-κB.[823-825] *Tax* results in an increase in free nuclear NF-κB and thereby increases expression from a number of cellular and viral genes under the influence of this transcriptional axis, including HIV-1.[826,827]

The *rex* protein appears to function similarly to the lentiviral *rev* protein, in that its expression results in the appearance of unspliced and singly spliced mRNA in the cytoplasm and the down-regulation of its own expression.[828-831] Also like *rev*, the target of *rex* is a complex RNA secondary structure; and although there is no obvious similarity in the *rex* binding site on the *Rex* Responsive Element (RxRE) to the *rev* binding site on RRE, *rex* is able to bind and transactive the HIV-1 RRE.[829,832] Several laboratories have recently demonstrated the *rex* binding site on the HIV-1 RRE lies outside of the *rev* binding site. Of note, the *rev* protein of HIV-1 cannot bind nor transactivate the RxRE.[828,833-835]

Finally, a recent report investigating the effect of integration site on expression of retroviral genes (as discussed in chapter 3) has implicated this mechanism as contributing to control of HTLV-I expression. Zoubak et al demonstrated that integration of HTLV-I proviruses into GC poor regions of the genome resulted in their transcriptional silence while integration into GC rich regions (which are maintained in a more open chromatin configuration) results in transcriptional activity.[836]

Despite these similarities in genomic organization and regulatory gene function, the fundamental pathological process in the generation of ATL by HTLV-I is different from the pathology resulting from HIV-1 infection. The leukemia/lymphoma resulting from HTLV-I infection is the product of a clonal expansion of a single infected cell.[837] The pathological process involved in the generation of the neuropathic disease associated with HTLV-I is insufficiently understood to make comparisons with HIV-1. It might be speculated, however, that the generation of ATL by HTLV-I is an incidental event in that the majority of infected people are asymptomatic and never develop malignancy despite a near lifelong infection; and that this incidental event is the result of integration into a sensitive region of the genome resulting in malignancy, as has been suggested for other oncogenic retroviruses. It might be further speculated, that HIV-1 has the same potential but that the relatively rapid development of immunodeficiency supersedes its oncogenic potential. Finally, if we exclude the relatively uncommon generation of malignancy, then HTLV-I infection is pathologically similar to SIV infection of either sooty mangabeys or African green monkeys or HIV-1 infection chimpanzees; that is, despite the ongoing low levels of viral replication, there is no apparent disease. Similarly, HTLV-II infection has not been associated with any disease despite its obvious maintenance within certain populations, demonstrating at least some level of retroviral replication. Finally, the evidence for the long-standing existence of HTLV-I like retroviruses within the human population (perhaps for centuries) might support the concept of an increased disease potential during the early course of interspecies transmission.[838]

HUMAN SPUMARETROVIRUS(ES) HSRV

Relatively little is known of this group of agents. Despite it being the first human retrovirus to be isolated, it has received little attention as a result of its lack of pathological potential. One immediately obvious feature of human spumaviruses which distinguish them from the other retroviruses considered herein is their relatively larger size, reaching close to 12 kilobases.[839,840] Despite this difference, there are a number of features which liken thenm to HIVs, SIVs and HTLVs. They undergo a complex pattern of mRNA splicing to yield their various structural and regulatory proteins; and they contain several multiply-spliced gene products derived from their 3' end which probably participate in HSRV transcriptional control.[76,839,841] There have been four potential gene products identified from these multiply-spliced mRNAs: (i) Bel-1; (ii) Bel-2; (iii) Bel-3; and (iv) Bet. Of these, only Bel-1's function has been firmly established and shown to be essential to the viral life cycle. This 36 kilodalton protein has been shown to be a *trans*-activator of transcription whose effects are mediated through two separate regions of the LTR located approximately 100 and 400 base pairs upstream of the transcriptional start site.[76,842-844] In addition to transactivating the HSRV LTR, there are two recent reports describing Bel-1's transactivation of the HIV-1 LTR; and unlike the *tax* transactivation of the HIV-1 LTR, Bel-1's target sequence is upstream of the NF-κB sites.[845,846] While there is much too little data available on HSRVs to date to make meaningful comparisons of their molecular biology to the other retroviruses discussed herein, they should provide another point along the spectrum of retroviral gene expression which will hopefully elucidate the host:virus interaction which allows the "peaceful co-existence" of retroviruses with their host.

REFERENCES

1. Hirsch VM, Dapolito GA, Goldstein S, McClure H, Emau P, Fultz PN, Isahakia M, Lenroot R, Myers G, Johnson PR. A distinct African lentivirus from Sykes' monkeys. J Virol 1993; 67:1517-1528.
2. Muller MC, Saksena NK, Nerrienet E, Chappey C, Herve VMA, Durand J-P, Legal-Campodonico P, Lang M-C, Digoutte J-P, Georges AJ, Georges-Courbot M-C, Sonigo P, Barre-Sinoussi F. Simian immunodeficiency viruses from Central and Western Africa: Evidence for a new species-specific lentivirus in Tantalus monkeys. J Virol 1993; 67:1227-1235.
3. Ohta Y, Masuda T, Tsujimoto H, Ishikawa K, Kodama T, Morikawa S, Nakai M, Honjo S, Hayami M. Isolation of simian immunodeficiency virus from African green monkeys and seroepidemiologic survey of the virus in various nonhuman primates. Int J Cancer 1988; 41:115-122.
4. Fukasawa M, Miura T, Hasegawa A, Morikawa S, Tsujimoto H, Miki K, Kitamura T, Hayami M. Sequence of simian immunodeficiency virus from African green monkeys a new member of the HIV/SIV group. Nature 1988; 333:457-461.
5. McClure MO The simian immunodeficiency viruses. Molec Aspects Med 1991; 12:247-253.
6. Fultz PN, McClure HM, Anderson DC, Swenson RB, Anand R, Srinivasan A. Isolation of a T-lymphocyte retrovirus from naturally infected sooty mangabey monkeys (*Cercocebus atys*). Proc Natl Acad Sci USA 1986; 83:5286-5290.
7. Marx PA, Li Y, Lerche NW, Sutjipto S, Gettie A, Yee JA, Brotman BH, Prince AM, Hanson A, Webster RG, Desrosiers RC. Isolation of a simian immunodeficiency virus related to human immunodeficiency virus type 2 from a West African pet sooty mangabey. J Virol 1991; 65:4480-4485.
8. Hirsch VM, Olmsted RA, Murphey-Corb M, Purcell RH, Johnson PR. An African lentivirus (SIVsm) closely related to HIV-2 Nature 1989; 339:389-392.
9. Gao F, Yue L, White AT, Pappas PG, Barchue J, Hanson AP, Greene BM, Sharp PM, Shaw GM, Hahn BH. Human infection by genetically diverse SIVsm-related HIV-2 in West Africa Nature 1992; 358:495-499.
10. Myers G, Pavlakis GN Evolutionary potential of complex retroviruses In: Levy J , ed, The Retroviridae. Plenum Press, New York, 1992:51-106.
11. Huet T, Chenyier R, Meyershans A, Roelants G, Wain-Hobson S. Genetic organization of a chimpanzee lentivirus related to HIV-1 Nature 1990; 345:356-358.
12. Peeters M, Honore C, Huet T, Bedjabaga L, Ossari S, Bussi P, Cooper CW, Delaporte E Isolation and partial characterization of an HIV-related virus occurring naturally in chimpanzees in Gabon. AIDS 1989; 3:625-630.

13. Francis D, Feorino P, Broderson J, McClure H, Getchell J, McGrath C, Swenson B, McDougal J, Palmer E, Harrison A, Barre-Sinoussi F, Chermann J-C, Montagnier L, Curran J, Cabradilla C, Kalyanaraman V. Infection of chimpanzees with lymphoadenopathy-associated virus. Lancet 1984; ii:1276-1277.

14. Alter H, Eichberg JW, Masur H, Saxinger W, Gallo R, Macher A, Lane H, Fauci A. Transmission of HTLV-III infection from human plasma to chimpanzees: an animal model for AIDS. Science 1984; 226:549-552.

15. Fultz P, McClure H, Swenson R, McGrath C, Brodie A, Getchell J, Jensen F, Anderson D, Brodson J, Francis D. Persistent infection of chimpanzees with human T-lymphotropic virus type III/lymphadenopathy-associated virus: a potential model for acquired immunodeficiency syndrome. J Virol 1986; 58:116-124.

16. Gadjusek D, Gibbs C, Rodgers-Johnson P, Amyx H, Asher D, Epstein L, Sarin P, Gallo R, Maluish A, Arthur L, Montagnier L, Mildvan D. Infection of chimpanzees by human T-lymphotropic retroviruses in brain and other tissue from AIDS patients. Lancet 1985; i:55-56.

17. Fultz P, McClure H, Swenson R, Anderson D HIV infection of chimpanzees as a model for testing chemotherapeutics. Intervirology 1989; 30:51-58.

18. Nara P, Robey W, Arthur L, Asher D, Wolff A, Gibbs CJ, Gajdusek D, Fischinger P. Persistent infection of chimpanzees with human immunodeficiency virus: serological responses and properties of reisolated viruses. J Virol 1987; 61:3173-3180.

19. Nara P, Smit L, Dunlop N, Hatch W, Merges M, Waters D, Kelliher J, Gallo R, Fischinger P, Goudsmit J. Emergence of viruses resistant to neutralization by V3-specific antibodies in experimental human immunodeficiency virus type 1 IIIB infection of chimpanzees. J Virol 1990; 64:3779-3791.

20. Bahraoui E, Yagello M, Billaud J, Sabatier J, Guy B, Muchmore E, Girard M, Gluckman J. Immunogenicity of the human immunodeficiency virus (HIV) recombinant nef gene product. Mapping of T-cell and B-cell epitopes in immunized chimpanzees. AIDS Res Hum Retroviruses 1990; 6:1087-1098.

21. Eichberg JW, Zarling JM, Alter HJ, Levy JA, Berman PW, Gregory T, Lasky LA, McClure J, Cobb KE, Moran PA, Hu SL, Kennedy RC, Chanh TC, Dreesman GR. T-cell responses to human immunodeficiency virus (HIV) and its recombinant antigens in HIV-infected chimpanzees. J Virol 1987; 61:3804-3808.

22. Zarling J, Eichberg J, Moran P, McClure J, Sridhar P, Hu S-L. Proliferative and cytoxic T cells to AIDS virus glycoproteins in chimpanzees immunized with a recombinant vaccinia virus expressing AIDS virus envelope glycoproteins. J Immunol 1987; 139:988-990.

23. Gojobori T, Moriyama EN, Ina Y, Ikeo K, Miura T, Tsujimoto H, Hayami M, Yokoyama S. Evolutionary origin of human and simian immunodeficiency viruses. Proc Natl Acad Sci USA 1990; 87:4108-4111.

24. Hirsch VM, Johnson PR. Pathogenesis of experimental SIV infection of macaques. Sem Virol 1992; 3:175-183.

25. Zhang Y-J, Ohman P, Putkonen P, Albert J, Walther L, Stalhandske P, Biberfeld G, Fenyo EM. Autologous neutralizing antibodies to SIVsm in

cynomologous monkeys correlates to prognosis. J Virol 1993; 197:609-615.

26. Khabbaz RF, Heneine W, George JR, Parekh B, Rowe T, Woods T, Switzer WM, McClure HM, Murphey-Corb M, Folks TM. Brief Report: Infection of a laboratory worker with simian immunodeficiency virus. N Engl J Med 1994; 330:172-177.

27. Novembre FJ, Johnson PR, Lewis MG, Anderson DC, Klumpp S, McClure HM, Hirsch VM. Multiple viral determinants contribute to pathogenicity of the acutely lethal simian immunodeficiency virus SIV_{smmPBj} variant. J Virol 1993; 67:2466-2474.

28. Israel ZR, Dean GA, Maul DH, O'Neil SP, Dreitz MJ, Mullins JI, Fultz PN, Hoover EA. Early pathogenesis of disease caused by $SIV_{smmPBj14}$ molecular clone 1.9 in macaques. AIDS Res Hum Retroviruses 1993; 9:277-286.

29. Fultz PN, Zack PM. Unique lentivirus-host interactions: $SIV_{smmPBj}14$ infection of macaques. Virus Res 1994; 32:205-225.

30. Rutherford GW, Lifson AR, Hessol NA, Darrow WW, O'Malley PM, Buchbinder SP, Barnhart JL, Bodecker TW, Cannon L, Doll LS, Holmberg SD, Harrison JS, Rogers. MF, Werdegar D, Jaffe HW. Course of HIV-1 infection in a cohort of homosexual and bisexual men: an 11 year follow up study. Br Med J 1990; 301:1183-1188.

31. Lifson AR, Buchbinder SP, Sheppard HW, Mawle AC, Wilber JC, Stanley M, Hart CE, Hessol NA, Holmberg SD. Long term human immunodeficiency virus infection in asymptomatic homosexual and bisexual men with normal CD4+ lymphocyte counts: Immunologic and virologic characteristics. J Infect Dis 1991; 163:959-965.

32. Sheppard HW, Lang W, Ascher MS, Vittinghoff E, Winkelstein W. The characterization of non-progressors: long term HIV-1 infection with stable CD4+ T-cell levels. AIDS 1993; 7:1159-1166.

33. Oka S, Ida S, Shioda T, Takebe Y, Kobayashi N, Shibuya Y, Ohyama K, Momota K, Kimura S, Shimada K. Genetic analysis of HIV-1 during rapid progression to AIDS in an apparently healthy man. AIDS Res Hum Retroviruses 1994; 10: 271-277.

34. Pedersen C, Lindhart BO, Jensen BL, Lauritzen E, Gerstoft J, Dickmeiss E, Gaub J, Scheibel E, Karlsmark T. Clinical course of primary HIV infection: consequences for subsequent course of infection. Br J Med 1989; 299:154-157.

35. DeCock KM, Adjorlolo G, Ekpini E, Sibailly T, Kouadio J, Maran M, Brattegaard K, Vetter KM, Doorly R, Gayle HD. Epidemiology and transmission of HIV-2: Why there is no HIV-2 pandemic. JAMA 1993; 270:2083-2086.

36. Weiss RA. Foamy retroviruses: A virus in search of a disease. Nature 1988; 333:497-498.

37. Mergia A, Luciw PA. Replication and regulation of primate foamy viruses. Virology 1991; 184:475-482.

38. Sugamura K, Hinuma Y. Human retroviruses: HTLV-I and HTLV-II. In: Levy, JA, ed. The Retroviradae. New York and London, Plenum Press 1992; 399-435.

39. Vallee H, Carre H. Sur la nature infectieuse de l'anemie du cheval. CR Hebd Seavc Acad Sci 1904; 139:331-333.

40. Charman HP, Bladen S, Gilden RV, Coggins L. Equine infectious anemia virus: evidence favoring classification as a retrovirus. J Virol 1976; 19:1073-1079.

41. Rous P. Comment. Proc Natl Acad Sci 58: 1967; 843-845.

42. Rous P. A sarcoma of the fowl transmissible by an agent separable from the tumor cells. J Exp Med 1911; 13: 397-411.

43. Little CC and Staff of Roscoe B Jackson Memorial Laboratory. The existence of non-chromosomal influence in the incidence of mammary tumors in mice. Science 1933; 78: 465-466.

44. Bittner JJ. Some possible effects of nursing on the mammary gland tumor incidence in mice. Science 1936; 84: 162.

45. Bittner JJ. The milk-influence of breast tumors in mice. Science 1942; 95:462-463.

46. Andervont HB, Bryan WR, Properties of the mouse mammary-tumor agent. J Natl Can Inst 1944; 5:143-149.

47. Lacassagne A. Apparition de cancers de la mammelle chez la souris male, soumise a des injections de folliculine. CR Acad Sci 1932; 195: 630-632.

48. Bittner JJ. Transfer of the agent for mammary cancer in mice by the male. 1952; Can Res 12: 387-397.

49. Gudnadottir M Visna-Maedi in sheep. Progr Med Virol 1974; 18:336-349.

50. Sigurdsson B, Palsson PA, Grimsson H. Visna a demyelinating transmissible disease of sheep. J Neuropath Exp Neurol 1957; 16:389-403.

51. Sigurdsson B, Palsson PA. Visna of sheep a slow demyelinating infection. Br J Exp Pathol 1958; 39:519-528.

52. Dungal N. Epizootic adenomatosis in the lungs of sheep. Its relation to verminous pneumonia and Jaagziekte. Proc Roy Soc Med 1938; 31:497-505.

53. Gislason G. Um maediveiki (Bunadarrit, Reykjavik, 1938)

54. Sigurdsson B, Thormar H, Palsson PA. Cultivation of visna virus in tissue culture. Arch ges Virusforsch 1960; 10: 368-381.

55. Rustigian R, Johnston P, Reihart H. Infection of monkey tissue cultures with virus-like agents. Proc Soc Exp Biol Med 1955; 88: 8-16.

56. Gajdusek DC, Rogers NG, Basnight M, Gibbs CJ, Jr, Alpers M. Transmission experiments with Kuru in chimpanzees and the isolation of latent viruses from the explanted tissues of affected animals. Ann NY Acad Sci 1969; 162:529-550.

57. Achong BG, Mansell PW, Epstein MA, Clifford P. An unusual virus in cultures from a human nasopharyngeal carcinoma. J Natl Cancer Inst 1971; 46:299-307.

58. Muller HK, Ball G, Epstein MA, Achong BG, Lenoir G, Levin A. The prevalence of naturally occurring antibodies to human syncytial virus in East African populations. J Gen Virol 1980; 47:399-406.

59. Temin H. RNA-dependent DNA polymerase in virions of Rous Sarcoma Virus. Nature 1970; 226, 1211-1213.

60. Baltimore D. RNA-dependent DNA polymerase in virions of RNA tumour viruses. Nature 1970; 226: 1209-1211.

61. Poiesz BJ, Ruscetti FW, Gazdar AF, Bunn PA, Minna JD, Gallo RC. Detection and isolation of type C retrovirus particles from fresh and cultured lymphocytes of a patient with cutaneous T-cell lymphoma. Proc

Natl Acad Sci USA 1980; 77:7415-7419.

62. Poiesz BJ, Ruscetti FW, Reitz MS, Kalyanaraman VS, Gallo RC. Isolation of a new type C retrovirus (HTLV) in primary uncultured cells of a patient with Sezary T-cell leukemia. Nature 1981; 294:268-271.

63. Chen ISY, McLaughlin J, Gasson JC, Clark SC, Golde DW. Molecular characterization of the genome of a novel human T-cell leukemia virus. Nature 1983; 305: 502-505.

64. Hjelle B, Mills R, Swenson S, Mertz G, Key C, Allen S. Incidence of hairy cell leukemia, mycosis fungoides, and chronic lymphocytic leukemia in first known HTLV-II endemic population. J Infect Dis 1991; 163:435-440.

65. Kalyanaraman VS, Narayanan R, Feorino P, Ramsey RB, Palmer EL, Chorba T, McDougal S, Getchell JP, Holloway B, Harrison AK, Cabradilla CD, Telfer M, Evatt B. Isolation and characterization of a human T cell leukemia virus type II from a hemophilia-A patient with pancytopenia. EMBO J 1985; 4:1455-1460.

66. Gottlieb MS, Schroff R, Schanker H, Weisman JD, Fan PT, Wolf RA, Saxon A. Pneumocystis carinii pneumonia and mucosal candidiasis in previously healthy homosexual men. N Engl J Med 1981; 305:1425-1430.

67. Gelmann EP, Popovic M, Blayney D, Masur H, Sidhu G, Stahl RE, Gallo RC. Proviral DNA of a retrovirus, Human T Cell Leukemia Virus, in two patients with AIDS. Science 1983; 220:862-865.

68. Essex M, McLane MF, Lee TH, Falk L, Howe CWS, Mullins JI, Cabradilla C, Francis DP. Antibodies to cell membrane antigens associated with Human T-Cell Leukemia Virus in patients with AIDS Science 1983; 220: 859-862.

69. Gallo RC, Salahudddin SZ, Popovic M, Shearer GM, Kaplan M, Haynes BF, Palker TJ, Redfield R, Oleske J, Safai B, White G, Foster P, Markham PD. Frequent detection and isolation of cytopathic retroviruses (HTLV-III) from patients with AIDS and at risk for AIDS. Science 1984; 224: 500-503.

70. Barre-Sinoussi F, Cherman JC, Rey F, Nugeyre MT, Chamaret S, Gruest J, Dauguet C, Axler-Blin C, Vezinet-Brun F, Rouzioux C, Rozenbaum W, Montagnier L. Isolation of a T-Lymphotropic retrovirus from a patient at risk for acquired immune deficiency syndrome (AIDS). Science 1983; 220:868-871.

71. Gallo RC, Sarin PS, Gelmann EP, Robert-Guroff M, Richardson E, Kalyanaraman VS, Mann D, Sidhu GD, Stahl RE, Zolla-Pazner S, Leibowitch J, Popovic M. Isolation of human T-Cell Leukemia Virus in acquired immune deficiency syndrome (AIDS). Science 1983; 220: 865-867.

72. Sarngadharan MG, Popovic M, Bruch L, Schupbach J, Gallo RC. Antibodies reactive with human T-lymphotropic retroviruses (HTLV-III) in the serum of patients with AIDS. Science 1984; 224: 506-508.

73. Popovic M, Sarngadharan MG, Read E, Gallo RC. Detection, isolation, continuous production of cytopathic retroviruses (HTLV-III) from patients with AIDS and Pre-AIDS. Science 1984; 224:497-500.

74. Schupbach J, Popovic M, Gilden RV, Gonda MA, Sarngadharan MG, GAllo RC. Serological analysis of a subgroup of Human T-Lymphocytropic retroviruses (HTLV-III) associated with AIDS. Science 1984; 224: 503-505.

75. Clavel F, Guetard D, Brun-Vezinet F, Chamaret S, Rey M-A, Santos-Ferreira MO, Laurent AG, Dauguet C, Katlama C, Rouzioux C, Klatzmann D, Champlimaud JL, Montagnier L. Isolation of a new human retrovirus from West African patients with AIDS. Science 1986; 233:343-346.

75a. Fultz PN, Gordon TP, Anderson DC, McClure HM. Prevalence of natural infection with simian immunodeficiency virus and simian T-cell leukemia virus type I in a breeding colony of sooty mangabey monkeys. AIDS 1990; 4:619-625.

76. Cullen BR. Regulatory proteins of complex retroviruses. Microbiol Rev 1992; 56:375-394.

77. Varmus H, Brown P. Retroviruses. In: Berg, Howe MM eds. Mobile DNA. Am. Soc. Microbiol, Washington DC, 1989:52-108

78. McCutchan JA. Medical aspects of the HIV epidemic. In: Morrow WJW, Haigwood NL ed. HIV Molecular Organization, Pathogenicity and Treatment. Elsevier Science Publishers B.V, 1993:1-28.

79. Weiss RA. How does HIV cause AIDS. Science 1993; 260:1273-1279.

80. Pantaleo G, Graziosi C, Fauci AS. The immunopathogenesis of human immunodeficiency virus infection. N Eng J Med 1993; 328:327-335.

81. Nelson JA, Reynolds-Kohler C, Oldstone MBA et al. HIV and HCMV coinfect brain cells in patients with AIDS. Virology 1988; 165:286-290.

82. Janeway C. Mls: makes a little sense. Nature 1991; 349:459-461.

83. Terai C, Kornbluth RS, Pauza CD et al. Apoptosis as a mechanism of cell death in cultured T lymphoblasts acutely infected with HINB-1. J Clin Invest 1991; 87:1710-1715.

84. Linette GP, Hartzman RJ, Ledbetter JA et al. HIV-1-infected T cells show a selective signaling defect after perturbation of CD3/antigen receptor. Science 1988; 241:573-576.

85. Duesberg PH. Human immunodeficiency virus and acquired immunodeficiency syndrome: correlation but not causation. Proc Natl Acad Sci USA 1989; 86:755.

86. Laurence J. Reservoirs of HIV infection or carriage: monocytic, dendritic, follicular dendritic, and B cells. Ann NY Acad Sci 1993; 693:52-64.

87. Gulizia J, Dempsey MP, Sharova N et al. Reduced nuclear import of human immunodeficiency virus type 1 preintegration complexes in the presence of a prototypic nuclear targeting signal. J Virol 1994; 68:2021-2025.

88. Bukrinsky MI, Sharova N, McDonald TL et al. Association of integrase, matrix, and reverse transcriptase antigens of human immunodeficiency virus type 1 with viral nucleic acids following acute infection. Proc Natl Acad Sci USA 1993; 90:6125-6129.

89. Bukrinsky MI, Sharova N, Dempsey MP et al. Active nuclear import of human immunodeficiency virus type 1 preintegration complexes. Proc Natl Acad Sci USA 1992; 89:6580-6584.

90. Lewis PF, Emerman M. Passage through mitosis is required for oncoretroviruses but not for the human immunodeficiency virus. J Virol 1994; 68:510-516.

91. Lewis P, Hensel M, Emerman M. Human immunodeficiency virus infection of cells arrested in the cell cycle. EMBO J 1992; 11:3053-3058.

92. Stevens SW, Griffith JD. Human immunodeficiency virus type 1 may

preferentially integrate into chromatin occupied by L1Hs repetitive elements. Proc Natl Acad Sci USA 1994; 91:5557-5561.

93. Pruss D, Bushman FD, Wolffe AP. Human immunodeficiency virus integrase directs integration to sites of severe DNA distortion within the nucleosome core. Proc Natl Acad Sci USA 1994; 91:5913-5917.

94. Milot E, Belmaaza A, Rassart E et al. Association of a host DNA structure with retroviral integration sites in chromosomal DNA. Virology 1994; 201:408-412.

95. Pryciak PM, Varmus HE. Nucleosomes, DNA-binding proteins, and DNA sequence modulate retroviral integration target site selection. Cell 1992; 69:769-780.

96. Pryciak PM, Muller H-P, Varmus HE. Simian virus 40 minichromosomes as targets for retroviral integration in vivo. Proc Natl Acad Sci USA 1992; 89:9237-9241.

97. Pryciak PM, Sil A, Varmus HE. Retroviral integration into minichromosomes in vitro. EMBO J 1992; 11:291-303.

98. Clark SJ, Saag MS, Decker WD et al. High titers of cytopathic virus in plasma of patients with symptomatic primary HIV-1 infection. N Engl J Med 1991; 324:954-960.

99. Daar ES, Moudgil T, Meyer RD et al. Transient high levels of viremia in patients with primary human immunodeficiency virus type 1 infection. N Engl J Med 1991; 324:961-964.

100. Coombs RW, Collier AC, Allain JP et al. Plasma viremia in human immunodeficiency virus infection. N Engl J Med 1989; 321:1626-1631.

101. Ho DD, Moudgil T, Alam M. Quantitation of human immunodeficiency virus type 1 in the blood of infected persons. N Engl J Med 1989; 321:1621-1625.

102. Koup RA, Safrit JT, Cao Y et al. Temporal association of cellular immune responses with the initial control of viremia in primary human immunodeficiency virus type 1 syndrome. J Virol 1994; 68:4650-4655.

103. Safrit JT, Andrews CA, Zhu T et al. Characterization of HIV-1 specific cytotoxic T lymphocyte clones isolated during acute seroconversion: recognition of autologous virus sequences within a conserved immunodominant epitope. J Exp Med 1994; 179:463-472.

104. Zhu T, Mo H, Wang N et al. Genotypic and phenotypic characterization of HIV-1 in patients with primary infection. Science 1993; 261:1179-1181.

105. Harper ME, Marselle LM, Gallo RC et al. Detection of lymphocytes expressing human T-lymphotrophic virus type III in lymph nodes and peripheral blood from infected individuals by in situ hybridization. Proc Natl Acad Sci USA 1986; 83:772-776.

106. Hsia K, Spector SA. Human immunodeficiency virus DNA is present in a high percentage of CD4+ lymphocytes of seropositive individuals. J Infect Dis 1991; 164:470-475.

107. Psallidopoulos MC, Schnittman SM, Thompson LM et al. Integrated proviral human immunodeficiency virus type 1 is present in CD4+ peripheral blood lymphocytes in healthy seropositive individuals. J Virol 1989; 63:4626-4631.

108. Schnittman SM, Psallidopoulos MC, Lane HC et al. The reservoir for HIV-1 in human peripheral blood is a T cell that maintains expression of

CD4. Science 1989; 245:305-308.

109. Poznansky MC, Walker B, Haseltine WA et al. A rapid method for quantitating the frequency of peripheral blood cells containing HIV-1 DNA. J Acq Imm Def Syndrome 1991; 4:368-373.

110. Connor RI, Mohri H, Cao Y et al. Increased viral burden and cytopathicity correlate temporally with CD4+ T-lymphocyte decline and clinical progression in human immunodeficiency virus type 1-infected individuals. J Virol 1993; 67:1772-1777.

111. Schnittman SM, Greenhouse JJ, Psallidopoulos MC et al. Increasing viral burden in CD4+ T cells from patients with human immunodeficiency virus (HIV) infection reflects rapidly progressive immunosuppression and clinical disease. Ann Int Med 1990; 113:438-443.

112. Bagnarelli P, Valenza A, Menzo S et al. Dynamics of molecular parameters of human immunodeficiency virus type 1 activity in vivo. J Virol 1994; 68: 2495-2502.

113. Bagasra O, Hauptman SP, Lischner HW et al. Detection of human immunodeficiency virus type 1 provirus in mononuclear cells by in situ polymerase chain reaction. N Engl J Med 1992; 326:1385-1391.

114. Embretson J, Zupancic M, Beneke J et al. Analysis of human immunodeficiency virus infected tissues by amplification and in situ hybridization reveals latent and permissive infections at single cell resolution. Proc Natl Acad Sci USA 1993; 90:357-361.

115. Embretson J, Zupancic M, Ribas JL et al. Massive covert infection of helper T lymphocytes and macrophages by HIV during the incubation period of AIDS. Nature 1993; 362:359-362.

116. Bagasra O, Seshamma T, Pomerantz RJ. Polymearase chain reaction in situ: intracellular amplification and detection of HIV-1 proviral DNA and other specific genes. J Immun Methods 1993; 158:131-145.

117. Bagasra O, Seshamma T, Oakes JW et al. High percentages of CD4-positive lymphocytes harbor the HIV-1 provirus in the blood of certain infected individuals. AIDS 1993; 7:1419-1425.

118. Lafeuillade A, Tamalet C, Pellegrino P et al. High viral burden in lymph nodes during early stages of HIV-1 infection. AIDS 1993; 11:1527-1528.

119. Pantaleo G, Graziosi C, Demarest JF et al. HIV infection is active and progressive in lymphoid tissue during the clinically latent stage of disease. Nature 1993; 362:355-358.

120. Patterson BK, Till M, Otto P et al. Detection of HIV-1 DNA and messenger RNA in individual cells by PCR-driven in situ hybridization and flow cytometry. Science 1993; 260:976-979.

121. Laughlin MA, Zeichner S, Kolson D et al. Sodium butyrate treatment of cells latently infected with HIV-1 results in the expression of unspliced viral RNA. Virology 1993; 196:496-505.

122. Folks TM, Justement J, Kinter A et al. Cytokine induced expression of HIV-1 in a chronically infected promonocytic cell line. Science 1987; 238:800-802.

123. Kinter AL, Poli G, Maury W et al. Direct and cytokine-mediated activation of protein kinase C induces human immunodeficiency virus expression in chronically infected promonocytic cells. J Virol 1990; 64:4306-4312.

124. Butera ST, Roberts BD, Lam L et al. Human immunodeficiency virus

type 1 RNA expression by four chronically infected cell lines indicates multiple mechanisms of latency. J Virol 1994; 68:2726-2730.

125. Folks TM, Clouse KA, Justement J et al. Tumor necrosis factor α induces expression of human immunodeficiency virus in a chronically infected T cell line clone Proc Natl Acad Sci USA 1989; 86:2365-2368.

126. Cannon P, Kim S-H, Ulich C et al. Analysis of *tat* function in human immunodeficiency virus type 1-infected low level expression cell lines U1 and ACH-2. J Virol 1994; 68:1993-1997.

127. Chen BK, Saksela K, Andino R et al. Distinct mode of human immunodeficiency virus type 1 proviral latency revealed by superinfection of nonproductively infected cell lines with recombinant luciferase-encoding viruses. J Virol 1994; 68:654-660.

128. Duan L, Oakes JW, Ferraro A et al. *Tat* and *Rev* differentially affect restricted replication of human immunodeficiency virus type 1 in various cells. Virology 1994; 199:474-478.

129. Winslows BJ, Pomerantz RJ, Bagosra O, Trono D. HIV-1 latency due to the site of proviral integration. Virology 1993; 196: 849-854.

130. Oakes JW, Bagasra O, Duan L et al. Alteration in nuclear factor-kB moieties are associated with HIV-1 proviral latency in certain monocytic cells. AIDS Res Human Retrov 1994; (in press).

131. Asjo B, Cefai D, Debre P et al. A novel mode of human immunodeficiency virus type 1 (HIV-1) activation: ligation of CD28 alone induces HIV-1 replication in naturally infected lymphocytes. J Virol 1993; 67:4395-4398.

132. Diegel ML, Moran PA, Gilliland LK et al. Regulation of HIV production by blood mononuclear cells from HIV infected donors: II. HIV-1 production depends on T-cell-monocyte interaction. AIDS Res Hum Retrov 1993; 9:465-473.

133. Moran PA, Diegel ML, Sias JC et al. Regulation of HIV production by blood mononuclear cells from HIV-infected donors: I. Lack of correlation between HIV-1 production and T cell activation. AIDS Res Hum Retrov 1993; 9:455-464.

134. Fraser JD, Irving BA, Crabtree GR, Weiss A. Regulation of IL-2 gene enhancer activity by the T cell accessory molecule CD28. Science 1991; 251:313-315.

135. Gendelman HE, Orenstein JM, Baca LM et al. The macrophage in the persistence and pathogenesis of HIV infection. AIDS 1989; 3:475-495.

136. Gartner S, Markovits P, Markovits DM et al. The role of mononuclear phagocytes in HTLV-III/LAV infection. Science 1986; 233:215-219.

137. Collman R, Godfrey B, Cutilli et al. Macrophage-tropic strains of human immunodeficiency virus type 1 utilize the CD4 receptor. J Virol 1990; 64:4468-4476.

138. Ho DD, Rota TR, Hirsch MS. Infection of monocyte/macrophages by human T-lymphotropic virus type III. J Clin Invest 1986; 77:1712-1714.

139. Gendelman HE, Narayan, Kennedy-Stoskopf S et al. Tropism of sheep lentiviruses from monocytes:susceptibility to infection and virus gene expression increase during maturation of monocytes to macrophages. J Virol 1986; 58:67-74.

140. Narayan O, Wolinsky JS, Clements JE et al. Slow virus replication: the role of macrophages in the persistence and expression of visna viruses of

sheep and goats. J Gen Virol 1982; 59:345-356.

141. Becker J, Ulrich P, Kunze R et al. Immunohistochemical detection of HIV structural proteins and distribution of T-lymphocytes and Langerhans cells in the oral mucosa of HIV infected patients. Virchows Arch Pathol Anat Histol 1988; 412:413-419.

142. Koenig S, Gendelman HE, Orenstein JM et al. Detection of AIDS virus in macrophaghes in brain tissue from AIDS patients with encephalopathy Science 1986; 233:1089-1093.

143. Pumarola-Sune T, Navia BA, Cordon-Cardo C. HIV antigen in the brains of patients with the AIDS dementia complex. Ann Neurol 1987; 21:490-496.

144. Rappersberger K, Gartner S, Schenk P et al. Langerhans cells are an actual site of HIV-1 replication. Intervirology 1988; 29:185-194.

145. Tenner-Racz K, Racz P, Bofill M et al. HTLV-III/LAV viral antigens in lymph nodes of homosexual men with persistent generalized lymphadopathy and AIDS. J Pathol 1986; 123:9-15.

146. Tschachler E, Groh V, Popovic M et al. Epidermal Langerhans cells: a target for HTLV-III/LAV infection. J Invest Dermatol 1987; 88:233-237.

147. Mikovits JA, Lohrey NC, Schulof R et al. Activation of infectious virus from latent human immunodeficiency virus infection of monocytes in vivo. J Clin Invest 1992; 90:1486-1491.

148. McElrath MJ, Steinman RM, Cohn ZA. Latent HIV-1 infection in enriched populations of blood monocytes and T cells from seropositive patients. J Clin Invest 1991; 87:27-30.

149. Rich EA, Chen ISY, Zack JA et al. Increased susceptibility of differentiated mononuclear phagocytes to productive infection with human immunodeficiency virus-1 (HIV-1). J Clin Invest 1992; 89:176-183.

150. Schrier RD, McCutchan JA, Wiley CA. Mechanisms of immune activation of human immunodeficiency virus in monocytes/macrophages. J Virol 1993; 67:5713-5720.

151. Schrier RD, McCutchan JA, Venable JC et al. T-cell induced expression of human immunodeficiency virus in macrophages. J Virol 1990; 64:3280-3288.

152. Fox CH, Tenner-Racz K, Racz P et al. Lymphoid germinal centers are reservoirs of human immunodeficiency virus type 1 RNA. J Infect Dis 1991; 164:1051-1057.

153. Fox CH, Hoover S, Currall VR et al. HIV in infected lymph nodes. Nature 1994; 370:256.

154. Zhang Y-M, Dawson SC, Landsman D et al. Persistence of four related human immunodeficiency virus subtypes during the course of zidovudine therapy: Relationship between virion RNA and proviral DNA. J Virol 1994; 68:425-432.

155. Michael NL, Chang G, Ehrenberg PK et al. HIV-1 proviral genotypes from the peripheral blood mononuclear cells of an infected patient are differentially represented in expressed sequences. J AIDS 1993; 6:1073-1085.

156. Greene WC. The molecular biology of human immunodeficiency virus type 1 infection. N Engl J Med 1991; 324:308-317.

157. Levy JA. Pathogenesis of human immunodeficiency virus infection. Microbiol Rev 1993; 57:183-289.

158. Vaishnav Y, Wong-Staal F. The biochemistry of AIDS. Annu Rev Biochem 1991; 60:578-630.

159. Bukrinsky MI, Sharova N, McDonald TL et al. Association of integrase, matrix, and reverse transcriptase antigens of human immunodeficiency virus type 1 with viral nucleic acids following acute infection. Proc Natl Acad Sci USA 1993; 90:6125-6129.

160. Sodroski JG, Rosen CA, Haseltine WA. Trans-acting transcriptional activation of the long terminal repeat of human T lymphocytropic viruses in infected cells. Science 1984; 225:381-385.

161. Sodroski JG, Rosen CA, Wong-Staal F et al. Trans-acting transcriptional regulation of human T-cell leukemia virus type III long terminal repeat. Science 1985; 227:171-173.

162. Atya SK, Guo C, Josephs SF et al. Trans-activator gene of human T lymphotropic virus type III (HTLVIII). Science 1985; 229:69-73.

163. Sodroski JG, Patarca R, Rosen CA et al. Location of the trans-activating region on the genome of human T-cell lymphotropic virus type III. Science 1985; 229:74-77.

164. Rosen CA, Sodroski, JG, Haseltine WA. Location of cis-acting regulatory sequences in the human T-cell lymphotropic virus type III (HTLVIII/LAV). Cell 1985; 41:813-823.

165. Cullen BR. Trans-activation of human immunodeficiency virus occurs via a bimodal mechanism. Cell 1986; 46:973-982.

166. Sheridan PL, Sheline CT, Milocco LH et al. *Tat* and the HIV-1 promoter: a model for RNA-mediated regulation of transcription. Seminars Virology 1993; 4:69-80.

167. Selby MJ, Bain ES, Luciw PA et al. Structure, sequence and position of the stem-loop structure in TAR determine transcriptional elongation by *tat* through the HIV-1 long terminal repeat. Genes Dev 1989; 3:547-558.

168. Kao S-Y, Calman A, Luciw PA et al. Antitermination of transcription within the long terminal repeat of HIV-1 by *tat* gene product. Nature 1987; 330:489-493.

169. Muesing MA, Smith DH, Capon DJ. Regulation of mRNA accumulation by a human immunodeficiency virus trans-activator protein. Cell 1987; 48: 691-701.

170. Peterlin BM, Luciw PA, Barr PJ et al. Elevated levels of mRNA can account for the trans-activation of human immunodeficiency virus. Proc Natl Acad Sci USA 1986; 83:9734-9738.

171. Sharp PA, Marciniak RA. HIV TAR: An RNA enhancer? Cell 1989; 59:229-230.

172. Colvin RA, Garcia-Blanco MA. Unusual structure of the human immunodeficiency virus Type 1 trans-activation response element. J Virol 1992; 66:930-935.

173. Selby MJ, Bain ES, Luciw PA. Structure, sequence and position of the stem-loop in TAR determine transcriptional elongation by *tat* through the HIV-1 long terminal repeat. Gene Dev 1989; 3:547-558.

174. Jakobovits A, Smith DH, Jakobovits EB et al. A discrete element 3' of human immunodeficiency virus (HIV-1) and HIV-2 mRNA initiation sites mediates transcriptional activation by an HIV trans-activator. Molec & Cell Biol 1988; 8:2555-2561.

175. Hauber J, Cullen BR. Mutational analysis of the trans-activation-responsive region of the human immunodeficiency virus type 1 long terminal repeat. J Virol 1988; 62:673-679.

176. Garcia JA, Harrich D, Soultanakis E et al. Human immunodeficiency virus type 1 LTR TATA and TAR region sequences required for transcriptional regulation. EMBO J 1989; 8:765-778.

177. Feng S, Holland EC. HIV-1 *tat* trans-activation requires the loop sequence within TAR. Nature 1988; 334:165-167.

178. Berkhout B, Silverman RH, Jeang K-T. *Tat* trans-activates the human immunodeficiency virus through a nascent RNA target. Cell 1989; 59:273-282.

179. Weeks KM, Ampe C, Schultz SC et al. Fragments of the HIV-1 *tat* protein specifically bind TAR RNA. Science 1990; 249:1281-1285.

180. Frankel AD, Biancalana S, Hudson D. Activity of synthetic peptides from the *tat* protein of human immunodeficiency virus type 1. Proc Natl Acad Sci USA 1989; 86:7397-7401.

181. Calnan BJ, Tidor B, Biancalana S et al. Arginine-mediated RNA recognition: the arginine fork. Science 1991; 252:1167-1171.

182. Calnan BJ, Biancalana S, Hudson D et al. Analysis of arginine rich peptides from the HIV *tat* protein reveqals unusual features of RNA-protein recognition. Genes Dev 1991; 5:201-210.

183. Cordingley MG, LaFemina RL, Callahan PL et al. Sequence specific interaction of *tat* protein and *tat* peptides with the transactivation responsive sequence element of human immunodeficiency virus type 1 in vitro. Proc Natl Acad Sci USA 1990; 87:8985-8989.

184. Loret EP, Georgel P, Johnson Jr. WC et al. Circular dichroism and molecular modeling yield a structure for the complex of human immunodeficiency virus type 1 trans-activation response RNA and the binding region of *tat*, the trans-acting transcriptional activator. Proc Natl Acad Sci USA 1992; 89:9734-9738.

185. Feng S, Holland E. HIV-1 *tat* trans-activation requires the loop sequence within TAR. Nature 1988; 334:165-167.

186. Berkout B, Jeang KT. Trans-activation of human immunodeficiency virus type 1 is sequence specific for both the single-stranded bulge and loop of the trans-acting responsive hairpin: a quantitative anlysis. J Virol 1989; 63:5501-5504.

187. Roy S, Parkin NT, Rosen C et al. Structural requirements for transactivation of human immunodeficiency virus type 1 long terminal repeat-directed gene expression by *tat*: importance of base pairing, loop sequence, and bulges in the *tat*-responsive sequence. J Virol 1990; 64:1402-1406.

188. Wu F, Garcia J, Sigman D et al. *Tat* regulates binding of the human immunodeficiency trans-acting region RNA loop-binding protein, TRP-185. Genes Dev 1991; 5:2128-2140.

189. Roy S, Agy M, Hovanessian AG et al. The integrity of the stem structure of human immunodeficiency virus type 1 *tat*-responsive sequence RNA is required for interaction with interferon-induced 68,000 M protein kinase. J Virol 1991; 65:632-640.

190. Alonso A, Derse D, Peterlin BM. Human chromosome 12 is required for optimal interactions between *tat* and TAR of human immunodeficiency virus type 1 in rodent cells. J Virol 1992; 66:4617-4621.

191. Madore SJ, Cullen BR. Genetic analysis of the cofactor requirement for human immunodeficiency virus type 1 *tat* function. J Virol 1993; 67:3703-3711.

192. Marciniak RA, Garcia-Blanco M, Sharp PA. Identification and characterization of a HeLa nuclear protein that specifically binds to the trans-activation-response (TAR) element of human immunodeficiency virus. Proc Natl Acad Sci USA 1990; 87:3624-3628.

193. Sharmeen L, Bass B, Sonenberg N et al. *Tat*-dependent adenosine-to-inosine modification of wild-type transactivation response RNA. Proc Natl Acad Sci USA 1991; 88:8096-8100.

194. Sheline C, Milocco L, Jones K. Two distinct nuclear transcription factors recognize loop and bulge residues of the HIV-1 TAR RNA hairpin. Genes Dev 1991; 5:2508-2520.

195. Kaczmarski W, Khan SA. Lupus autoantigen KU protein binds HIV-1 TAR RNA in vitro. Biochem Biophys Res Comm 1993; 196:935-942.

196. Sullenger BA, Gallardo HF, Ungers GE et al. Over-expression of TAR sequences renders cells resistant to human immunodeficiency virus replication. Cell 1990; 63:601-608.

197. Sullenger BA, Gallardo HF, Ungers GE et al. Analysis of trans-acting response decoy RNA-mediated inhibition of human immunodeficiency virus type 1 transactivation. J Virol 1991; 65:6811-6816.

198. Newstein M, Stanbridge EJ, Casey G et al. Human chromosome 12 encodes a species-specific factor which increases human immunodeficiency virus type 1 *tat*-mediated trans-activation in rodent cells. J Virol 1990; 64:4565-4567.

199. Hart CE, Ou C-Y, Galphin JC et al. Human chromosome 12 is required for elevated HIV-1 expression in human-hamster hybrid cells. Science 1989; 246:488-491.

200. Selby MJ, Peterlin BM. Transactivation by HIV-1 *tat* via a heterologous RNA binding protein. Cell 1990; 62:769-776.

201. Southgate C, Zapp ML, Green MR. Activation of transcription by HIV-1 *tat* protein tethered to nascent RNA through another protein. Nature 1990; 345:640-642.

202. Tiley LS, Madore SJ, Malim MH et al. The VP-16 transcription activation domain is functional when targeted to a promoter-proximal RNA sequence. Genes Develop 1992; 5:2077-2087.

203. Newstein M, Lee I-S, Venturini DS et al. A chimeric human immunodeficiency virus type 1 TAR region which mediates high level trans-activation in both rodent and human cells. Virology 1993; 197:825-828.

204. Cullen BR. Does HIV-1 *Tat* induce a change in viral initiation rights? Cell 1993; 73:417-420.

205. Wright CM, Felber BK, Paskalis H et al. Expression and characterization of the trans-activator of HTLV-III/LAV virus. Science 1986; 234:988-992.

206. Peterlin BM, Luciw PA, Barr PJ et al. Elevated levels of mRNA can account for the trans-activation of human immunodeficiency virus. Proc Natl Acad Sci USA 1986; 83:9734-9738.

207. Cullen BR. The HIV-1 *tat* protein: An RNA sequence specific processivity factor? Cell 1990; 63:655-657.

208. Laspia MF, Rice AP, Mathews MB. HIV-1 *Tat* protein increases tran-

scriptional initiation and stabilizes elongation. Cell 1990; 59:283-292.

209. Laspia MF, Rice AP, Mathews MB. Synergy between HIV-1 *Tat* and adenovirus E1a is principally due to stabilization of transcriptional elongation. Genes Develop 1990; 4:2397-2408.

210. Marciniak RA, Sharp PA. HIV-1 *tat* protein promotes formation of more-processive elongation complexes. EMBO J 1991; 10:4189-4196.

211. Lu X, Welsh TM, Peterlin BM. The human immunodeficiency virus type 1 long terminal repeat specifies two different transcription complexes, only one of which is regulated by *tat*. J Virol 1993; 67:1752-1760.

212. Berkhout B, Jeang K-T. Functional roles for the TATA promoter and enhancers in basal and *tat*-induced expression of the human immunodeficiency virus type 1 long terminal repeat. J Virol 1992; 66:139-149.

213. Ratnasabapathy R, Sheldon M, Johal L, Hernandez N. The HIV-1 long terminal repeat contains an unusual element that induces the synthesis of short RNAs from various mRNA and snRNA promoters. Genes Dev 1990; 4:2061-2074.

214. Sheldon M, Ratnasabapathy R, Hernandez N. Characterization of the inducer of short transcripts a human immunodeficiency virus type 1 transcriptional element that activates the synthesis of short RNAs Molec Cell Biol 1993; 13:1251-1263.

215. Rougvie AE, Lis JT. The RNA polymerase II molecule at the 5' end of the uninduced hsp70 gene of D. melanogaster is transcriptionally engaged. Cell 1988; 54:795-804.

216. Adams M, Sharmeen L, Kimpton J, Romeo JM, Garcia JV, Peterlin BM, Groudine M, Emerman M. Cellular latency in human immunodeficiency virus-infected individuals with high CD4 levels can be detected by the presence of promoter-proximal transcripts. Proc Natl Acad Sci USA 1994; 91:3862-3866.

217. Kato H, Sumimoto H, Pognonec P, Chen C-H, Rosen CA, Roeder RG. HIV-1 *tat* acts as a processivity factor in vitro in conjunction with cellular elongation factors. Genes Develop 1992; 6:655-666.

218. Flores O, Maldonado E, Reinberg D. Factors involved in specific transcription by mammalian polymerase II: Factors IIE and IIF independently interact with RNA polymerase II. J Biol Chem 1989; 264:8913-8921.

219. Flores O, Ha I, Reinberg D. Factors involved in specific transcription by mammalian RNA polymerase II. J Biol Chem 1990; 265:5629-5634.

220. Kitajima S, Tanaka Y, Kawaguchi T, Nagaoka T, Weissman SM, Yasukochi Y. A heteromeric transcription factor required for mammalian RNA polymerase II. Nucl Acid Res 1990; 18: 4843-4849.

221. Reinberg D, Roeder RG. Factors involved on specific transcription by mammalian RNA polymerase II. J Biol Chem 1987; 262:3331-3337.

222. Kamine J, Subramanian T, Chinnadurai G. Sp-1 dependent activation of a synthetic promoter by human immunodeficiency virus type 1 *tat* protein. Proc Natl Acad Sci USA 1991; 88:8510-8514.

223. Southgate CD, Green MR. The HIV-1 *tat* protein activates transcription from an upstream DNA-binding site: implications for *tat* function. Genes Develop 1991; 5:2496-2507.

224. Kamine J, Subramanian T, Chinnadurai G. Activation of a heterologous promoter by human immunodeficiency virus type 1 *tat* requires Sp-1 and is distinct from the mode of activation by acidic transcriptional activa-

tors. J Virol 1993; 67:6828-6834.

225. Ghosh S, Selby MJ, Peterlin BM. Synergism between *tat* and VP16 is trans-activation of HIV-1 LTR. J Molec Biol 1993; 234:610-619.

226. Olsen HS, Rosen CA. Contribution of the TATA motif to *tat*-mediated transcriptional activation of human immunodeficiency virus gene expression. J Virol 1992; 66:5594-5597.

227. Jeang K-T, Berkhout B. Kinetics of HIV-1 long terminal repeat transactivation: Use of intragenic robozyme to assess rate-limiting steps. J Biol Chem 1992; 267:17891-17899.

228. Taylor JP, Pomerantz RJ, Bagasra O, Chowdhury M, Rappaport J, Khalili K, Amini S. TAR-independent transactivation by *tat* in cells derived from the CNS: a novel mechanism of HIV-1 gene regulation. EMBO J 1992; 11:3395-3403.

229. Harrich D, Garcia J, Mitsuyasu R, Gaynor R. TAR independent activation of the human immunodeficiency virus in phorbol ester stimulated T lymphocytes. EMBO J 1990; 9:4417-4423.

230. Taylor JP, Pomerantz RJ, Raj GV, Kashanchi F, Brady JN, Amini S, Khalili K. Central nervous system-derived cells express a κB-binding activity that enhances human immunodeficiency virus type 1 transcription in vitro and facilitates TAR-independent transactivation by *tat*. J Virol 1994; 68:3971-3981.

231. Bagasra O, Khallili K, Seshamma T, Taylor J, Pomerantz R. TAR-independent replication of human immunodeficiency virus type 1 in glial cells. J Virol 1992; 66:7522-7528.

232. Berkhout B, Gatignol A, Rabson AB, Jeang K-T. TAR-independent activation of the HIV-1 LTR: evidence that *tat* requires specific regions of the promoter. Cell 1990; 62:757-767.

233. Cullen BR. Mechanism of action of regulatory proteins encoded by complex retroviruses. Microb Rev 1992; 56:375-394.

234. Braddock M, Chambers A, Wilson W, Esnouf MP, Adams SE, Kingsman AJ, Kingsman SM. HIV-1 *tat* "activate" presynthesized RNA in the nucleus. Cell 1989; 58:269-279.

235. Braddock M, Chambers A, Wilson W, Esnouf MP, Adams SE, Kingsman AJ, Kingsman SM. HIV-1 *tat* "activates" presynthesized RNA in the nucleus. Cell 1989; 58:269-279.

236. Braddock M, Cannon P, Muckenthaler M, Kingsman AJ, Kingsman SM. Inhibition of human immunodeficiency virus type 1 *tat*-dependent activation of translation in Xenopus oocytes by the benzodiazepine R024-7429 requires trans-activation response element loop sequences. J Virol 1994; 68:25-33.

237. Feinberg MB, Jarrett RF, Aldovini A, Gallo RC, Wong-Staal F. HTLV-III expression and production involve complex regulation at the levels of splicing and translation of viral RNA. Cell 1986; 46:807-817.

238. Rosen CA, Sodroski JG, Goh WC, Dayton AI, Lippke J, Haseltine WA. Post-transcriptional regulation accounts for trans-activation of human T-lymphotropic virus type III. Nature 1986; 319:555-559.

239. Wright CM, Felber BK, Paskalis H, Pavlakis GN. Expression and characterization of the trans-activator of HTLV-III/LAV virus. Science 1986; 234:988-992.

240. Rice AP, Mathews MB. Transcriptional but not translational regulation

of HIV-1 by the *tat* gene product. Nature 1988; 332:551-553.

241. Sadaie M, Benter T, Wong-Staal F. Site-directed mutagenesis of two trans-regulatory genes (tatIII,trs) of HIV-1. Science 1988; 239:91-913.

242. Garcia J, Harrich D, Soultanakis E, Wu F, Mitsuyasu R, Gaynor R. Functional domains required for *tat*-induced transcriptional activation of the HIV-1 long terminal repeat. EMBO J 1988; 8:765-778.

243. Kuppuswamy M, Subramanain T, Srinivasan A, Chinnadurai G. Multiple functional domains of *tat*, the trans-activator of HIV-1, defined by mutational analysis. Nucl Acids Res 1989; 17:3551-3561.

244. Tiley LS, Brown PH, Cullen BR. Does the human immunodeficiency virus *tat* transactivator contain a discrete activation domain? Virology 1990; 178:560-567.

245. Rice AP, Carlotti F. Mutational analysis of the conserved cysteine rich region of the human immunodeficiency virus type 1 *tat* protein. J Virol 1990; 64:1864-1868.

246. Rice AP, Carlotti F. Structural analysis of wild type and mutant human immuynodeficiency virus type 1 *tat* proteins J Virol 1990; 64:6018-6026.

247. Hauber J, Malim MH, Cullen BR. Mutational analysis of the conserved basic domain of human immunodeficiency virus *tat* protein J Virol 1989; 63:1181.

248. Ruben S, Perkins A, Purcell R, Joung K, Sia R, Burghoff R, Haseltine WA, Rosen CA. Structural and functional characterization of human immunodeficiency virus *tat* protein. J Virol 1989; 63:1-8.

249. Sadai MR, Rappaport J, Benter T, Josephs SF, Willis R, Wong-Staal F. Missense mutations in an infectious human immunodeficiency viral genome: functional mapping of *tat* and identification of the *rev* splice acceptor. Proc Natl Acad Sci USA 1988; 85:9224-9228.

250. Siegal LJ, Ratner L, Josephs SF, Derse D, Feinberg MB, Reyes GA, O'Brien SJ, Wong-Staal F. Transactivation induced by human T-lymphotrophic virus type III (HTLV-III) maps to a viral sequence encoding 58 amino acids and lacks tissue specificity. Virology 1986; 48:226-231.

251. Garcia JA, Harrich D, Pearson L, Mitsuyasu R, Gaynor RB. Functional domains required for *tat*-induced transcriptional activation of the HIV-1 long terminal repeat. EMBO J 1988; 7:3143-3147.

252. Rappaport J, Lee SJ, Khalili K, Wong-Staal F. The acidic amino-terminal region of the HIV-1 *tat* protein constitutes an essential activating domain. New Biol 1989; 1:101-110.

253. Subramanian T, D'Sa-Eipper C, Elangovan B, Chinnadurai G. The activation region of the *tat* protein of human immunodeficiency virus type-1 functions in yeast. Nucl Acid Res 1994; 22:1496-1499.

254. Carroll R, Martarano L, Derse D. Identification of lentivirus *tat* functional domains through generation of equine infectious anemia virus/human immunodeficiency virus type 1 *tat* gene chimeras. J Virol 1991; 65:3460-3467.

255. Derse D, Carvalho M, Carroll R, Peterlin BM. A minimal lentivirus *tat*. J Virol 1991; 65:7012-7015.

256. Weeks KM, Crothers DM. RNA recognition by *tat*-derived peptides: interaction in the major groove? Cell 1991; 66:577-588.

257. Siomi H, Shida H, Maki M, Hatanaka M. Effects of a highly basic re-

gion of human immunodeficiency virus *tat* protein on nucleolar localization. J Virol 1990; 64:1803-1807.

258. Sumner-Smith M, Roy S, Barnett R, Reid LS, Kuperman R, Delling U, Sonenberg N. Critical chemical features in trans-acting-responsive RNA are required for interaction with human immunodeficiency virus type 1 *tat* protein. J Virol 1991; 65:5196-5202.

259. Churcher MJ, Lamont C, Hamy F, Dingwall C, Green SM, Lowe AD, Butler JG, Gait MJ, Karn J. High affinity binding of TAR RNA by the human immunodeficiency virus type 1 *tat* protein requires base-pairs in the RNA stem and amino acid residues flanking the basic region. J Molec Biol 1993; 230:90-110.

260. Weeks KM, Crothers DM. RNA binding assays for *tat*-derived peptides: Implications for specificity. Biochem 1992; 31:10281-10287.

261. Jeang K-T, Berkhout B, Dropulic B. Effects of integration and replication on transcription of the HIV-1 long terminal repeat. J Biol Chem 1993; 33:24940-24949.

262. Kessler M, Mathews MB. *Tat* transactivation of the human immunodeficiency virus type 1 promoter is influenced by basal promoter activity and the simian virus 40 origin of DNA replication. Proc Natl Acad Sci USA 1991; 88:10018-10022.

263. Vives E, Charneau P, van Rietschoten J, Rochat H, Bahraoui E. Effects of the *tat* basic domain on human immunodeficiency virus type 1 transactivation, using chemically synthesized *tat* protein and *tat* peptides. J Virol 1994; 68:3343-3353.

264. Jeyapaul J, Reddy MR, Khan SA. Activity of synthetic *tat* peptides in human immunodeficiency virus type 1 long terminal repeat-promoted transcription in a cell free system. Proc Natl Acad Sci USA 1990; 87:7030-7034.

265. Green M, Lowenstein P. Autonomous functional domains of chemically synthesized human immunodeficiency virus *tat* transactivator protein. Cell 1988; 55:1179-1188.

266. Modesti N, Garcia J, Debouck C, Peterlin M, Gaynor R. Trans-dominant *tat* mutants with alterations in the basic domain inhibit HIV-1 gene expression. New Biol 1991; 3:759-768.

267. Pearson L, Garcia J, Wu F, Modesti N, Nelson J, Gaynor R. A transdominant *tat* mutant that inhibits *tat*-induced gene expression from the human immunodeficiency virus long terminal repeat. Proc Natl Acad Sci USA 1990; 87:5079-5083.

268. Sheline C, Milocco L, Jones K. Two distinct nuclear transcription factors recognize loop and bulge residues of the HIV-1 TAR RNA hairpin. Genes Dev 1991; 5:2508-2520.

269. Marciniak RA, Calnan BJ, Frankel AD, Sharp PA. HIV-1 *tat* protein transactivates transcription in vitro. Cell 1990; 63:791-802.

270. Marciniak RA, Garcia-Blanco MA, Sharp PA. Identification and characterization of a HeLa nuclear protein that specifically binds to the transactivation respons (TAR) element of human immunodeficiency virus. Proc Natl Acad Sci USA 1990; 87:3624-3628.

271. McCormack SJ, Thomas DC, Samuel CE. Mechanism of interferon action: identification of a RNA binding domain within the N-terminal region of the human RNA dependent P1/eIF-2 alpha protein kinase. Virol-

ogy 1992; 188:47-56.

272. Rounesville MP, Kumar A. Binding of a host cell nuclear protein to the stem region of human immunodeficiency virus type 1 trans-activation-responsive RNA. J Virol 1992; 66:1688-1694.

273. Jeang K-T, Chun R, Lin NH, Gatignol A, Glabe CG, Fan H. In vitro and in vivo binding of human immunodeficiency virus type 1 *tat* protein and Sp-1 transcription factor. J Virol 1993; 67:6224-6233.

274. Herrmann CH, Rice AP. Specific Interaction of the human immunodeficiency virus *tat* proteins with cellular protein kinase. Virology 1993; 197:601-608.

275. Jakobovits A, Rosenthal A, Capon DJ. Trans-activation of HIV-1 LTR-directed gene expression by *tat* requires protein kinase C. EMBO J 1990; 9:1165-1170.

276. Aso T, Vassavada H, Kawaguchi T, Germino F, Ganguly S, Kitajima S, Weissman S, Yasukochi Y. Characterization of cDNA from the large subunit of the transcription initiation factor TFIIF. Nature 1992; 355:461-464.

277. Finkelstein A, Kostrub C, Li J, Chavez D, Wang B, Fang S, Greenblatt J, Burton Z. A cDNA encoding RAP74 a general initiation factor for transcription by RNA polymerase II. Nature 1992; 355:464-467.

278. Nelbock P, Dillon R, Perkins A, Rosen CA. A cDNA for a protein that interacts with the human immunodeficiency virus *tat* transactivator. Science 1990; 248:1650-1653.

279. Ohana B, Moore PA, Ruben SM, Southgate CD, Green MR, Rosen CA. The type 1 human immunodeficiency virus *tat* binding protein is a transcriptional activator belonging to an additional family of evolutionarily conserved genes. Proc Natl Acad Sci USA 1993; 90:138-142.

280. Shibuya H, Irie K, Ninomiya-Tsuji J, Goebl M, Taniguchi T, Matsumoto K. New human gene encoding a positive modulator of HIV *tat*-mediated transactivation. Nature 1992; 357:700-702.

281. Swafield JC, Bromberg JF, Johnston SA. Alterations in a yeast protein resembling HIV *tat*-binding protein relieve requirement for an acidic activation domain in GAL4. Nature 1992; 357:698-700.

282. Gait MJ, Karn J. RNA recognition by the human immunodeficiency virus *tat* and *rev* proteins. TIBS 1993; 18:255-259.

283. Parslow TG. Human Retroviruses. In: Cullen BR, ed. Frontiers in Molecular Biology 1993:101-136.

284. Guatelli JC, Gingeras TR, Richman DD. Alternative splice acceptor utilization during human immunodeficiency virus type 1 infection of cultured cells. J Virol 1990; 64: 4093.

285. Robert-Guroff M, Popovic M, Gartner S, Markham P, Gallo RC, Reitz MS. Structure and expression of *tat-*, *rev*, and nef-specific transcripts of human immunodeficiency virus type 1 in infected lymphocytes and macrophages. J Virol 1990; 64:3391-3398.

286. Schwartz S, Felber BK, Benko DM, Fenyo EM, Pavlakis GN. Cloning and functional analysis of multiply-spliced mRNA species of human immunodeficiency virus type 1. J Virol 1990; 64:2519-2529.

287. Schwartz S, Felber BK, Fenyo EM, Pavlakis GN. Env and Vpu proteins of human immunodeficiency virus type are produced from multiple bicistronic mRNAs. J Virol 1990; 64:5448-5456.

288. Schwartz S, Felber BK, Pavlakis GN. Mechanism of translation of monocistronic and multicistronic human immunodeficiency virus type 1 mRNAs. Molec Cell Biol 1992; 12:207-219.

289. Purcell DFJ, Martin MA. Alternative splicing of human immunodeficiency virus type 1 mRNA modulates viral protein expression, replication and infectivity. J Virol 1993; 67:6365-6378.

290. Padgett RA, Grabowski PJ, Konarska MM, Seiler SR, Sharp PA. Splicing of messenger RNA precursors. Annu Rev Biochem 1986; 55:1119-1150.

291. Green MR. Biochemical mechanisms of constitutive and regulated pre-mRNA splicing. Annu Rev Cell Biol 1991; 7:559-599.

292. Feinberg MB, Jarrett RF, Aldovini A, Ballo RC, Wong-Staal F. HTLV-III expression and production involve complex regulation at the levels of splicing and translation of viral RNA. Cell 1986; 46, 807-817.

293. Sodroski J, Goh WC, Rosen C, Dayton A, Terwilliger E, Haseltine W. A second post-transcriptioanl trans-activator gene required for HTLV-III replication. Nature 1986; 321: 412-417.

294. Felber BK, Hadzopoulou-Cladaras M, Cladaras D, Copeland T, Pavlakis GN. *Rev* protein of human immunodeficiency virus type 1 affects the stability and transport of the viral mRNA. Proc Natl Acad Sci USA 1989; 86:1495-1499.

295. Emerman M, Vazeux R, Peden K. The *rev* gene product of the human immunodeficiency virus affects envelope specific RNA localization. Cell 1989; 57:1155.

296. Hammarskjold M-L, Heimer J, Hammarskjold B, Sangwan I, Albert L, Rekosh D. Regulation of human immunodeficiency virus env expression by the *rev* gene product. J Virol 1989; 63:1959-1966.

297. Malim MH, Hauber J, Le S-Y, Maizel JV, Cullen BR. The HIV-1 *rev* trans-activator acts through a structured target sequence to activate nuclear export of unspliced viral mRNA Nature 1989; 338:254-257.

298. Terwilliger E, Burghoff R, Sia R, Sodroski J, Haseltine W, Rosen C. The art gene product of human immunodeficiency virus is required for replication. J Virol 1988; 62:655-658.

299. Pomerantz RJ, Seshamma T, Trono D. Efficient replication of human immunodeficiency virus type 1 requires a threshold level of *Rev*: Potential implications for latency. J Virol 1992; 66:1809-1813.

301. Dayton AI, Terwilliger EF, Potz J, Kowalski M, Sodroski JG, Haseltine WA. Cis-acting sequences responsive to the *rev* gene product of the human immunodeficiency virus. J AIDS 1988; 1:441-452.

302. Hadzopoulou-Cladaras M, Felber BK, Cladaras C, Athanassopoulos A, Tse A, Pavlakis GN The *rev* (trs/art) protein of human immunodeficiency virus type 1 affects viral mRNA and protein expression via a cis-acting sequence in the env region. J Virol 1989; 63:1265-1274.

303. Cochrane AW, Chen C-H, Rosen CA. Specific interaction of the human immunodeficiency virus *rev* protein with a structured region in the env mRNA. Proc Natl Acad Sci USA 1990; 87:1198-1202.

304. Daeffler S, Klotman ME, Wong-Staal F. Trans-activating *rev* protein of the human immunodeficiency virus type 1 interacts directly and specifically with its target RNA. Proc Natl Acad Sci USA 1990; 87:4571-4575.

305. Kjems J, Brown M, Chang DD, Sharp PA. Structural analysis of the interaction between the human immunodeficiency virus *rev* protein and the

rev response element. Proc Natl Acad Sci USA 1991; 88:683-687.

306. Malim MH, Tiley LS, McCarn DF, Rusche JR, Hauber J, Cullen BR. HIV-1 structural gene expression requires binding of the *rev* trans-activator to its RNA target sequences. Cell 1990; 60:675-683.

307. Heaphy S, Dingwall C, Ernberg I, Gait MJ, Green SM, Karn J, Lowe AD, Singh M, Skinner MA. HIV-1 regulator of virion expression (*Rev*) protein binds to an RNA stem-loop structure located within the *rev* response element region. Cell 1990; 60:685-693.

308. Daly TJ, Cook KS, Gray GS, Maione TE, Rusche JR. Specific binding of HIV-1 recombinant *rev* protein to the *rev*-responsive element in vitro. Nature 1989; 342:816-819.

309. Le S-Y, Malim MH, Cullen BR, Maizel JV. A highly conserved RNA folding region coincident with the *rev* response element of primate immunodeficiency viruses. Nucl Acid Res 1990; 18:1613-1623.

310. Holland SM, Ahmad N, Maitra RK, Wingfield P, Venkatesan S. Human immunodeficiency virus *rev* protein recognizes a target sequence in *rev*-responsive element RNA within the context of RNA secondary structure. J Virol 1990; 64:5966-5975.

311. Olsen HS, Nelbock P, Cochrane AW, Rosen CA. Secondary structure is the major determinant for interaction of HIV *rev* protein with RNA. Science 1990; 247:845-848.

312. Dayton ET, Powell DM, Dayton AI. Functional analysis of CAR, the target sequence for the *rev* protein of HIV-1. Science 1989; 246:1625-1629.

313. Huang X, Hope TJ, Bond BL, McDonald D, Grahl K, Parslow TG. Minimal *rev*-response element for type 1 human immunodeficiency virus. J Virol 1991; 65:2131-2134.

314. Bartel DP, Zapp ML, Green MR, Szostak JW. HIV-1 *rev* regulation involves recognition of non-Watson-Crick base pairs in viral RNA. Cell 1991; 67:529-536.

315. Dayton ET, Konings DAM, Powell DM, Shapiro BA, Butini L, Maizel JV, Dayton AI. Extensive sequence-specific information throughout the CAR/RRE, the target sequence of the human immunodeficiency virus type 1 *rev* protein. J Virol 1992; 66:1139-1151.

316. Cook KS, Fisk GJ, Hauber J, Usman N, Daly TJ, Rusche JR. Characterization of HIV-1 *rev* protein: binding stoichiometry and minimal RNA substrate. Nucl Acid Res 1991; 19:1577-1583.

317. Tiley LS, Malim MH, Tewary HK, Stockley PG, Cullen BR. Identification of a high affinity RNA-binding site for the human immunodeficiency virus type 1 *rev* protein. Proc Natl Acad Sci USA 1992; 89:758-762.

318. Bogerd H, Greene WC. Dominant negative mutants of HTLV-I *Rex* and HIV-1 *Rev* fail to multimerize in vivo. J Virol 1993; 67:2496-2502.

319. Madore SJ, Tiley LS, Malim MH, Cullen BR. Sequence requirements for *rev* multimerization in vivo. Virology 1994; 202:186-194.

320. Cole JL, Gehman JD, Shafer JA, Kuo LC. Solution oligomerization of the *rev* protein of HIV-1: Implications for function. Biochem 1993; 32:11769-11775.

321. Daly TJ, Doten RC, Rennert P, Auer M, Jaksche H, Donner A, Fisk G, Rusche JR. Biochemical characterization of binding of multiple HIV-1 *rev* monomeric proteins to the *rev* responsive element. Biochem 1993;

32:10497-10505.

322. Cullen BR, Hauber J, Campbell K, Sodroski JG, Haseltine WA, Rosen CA. Subcellular localization of the human immunodeficiency virus trans-acting art gene product. J Virol 1988; 62:2498-2501.

323. Hope TJ, Huang X, McDonald D, Parslow TG. Steroid-receptor fusion of the HIV-1 *rev* transactivator: mapping cryptic functions of the arginine-rich motif. Proc Natl Acad Sci USA 1990; 87:7787-7791.

324. Kalland KH, Szilvay AM, Langhoff E, Haukenes G. Subcellular distribution of human immunodeficiency virus type 1 *rev* and colocalization of *rev* with RNA splicing factors in a speckled pattern in the nucleoplasm. J Virol 1994; 68:1475-1485.

325. Chang DD, Sharp PA. Regulation by HIV *rev* depends upon recognition of splice sites. Cell 1989; 59:789-795.

326. Staffa A, Cochrane A. The *tat/rev* intron of human immunodeficiency virus type 1 is inefficiently spliced because of suboptimal signals in the 3' splice site. J Virol 1994; 68:3071-3079.

327. Hammarskjold M-L, Li H, Rekosh D, Prasad S. Human immunodeficiency virus env expression becomes *rev*-independent if the env region is not defined as an intron. J Virol 1994; 68:951-958.

328. Nasioulas G, Zolotukhin AS, Tabernero C, Solomin L, Cunningham CP, Pavlakis GN, Felber BK. Elements distinct from human immunodeficiency virus type 1 splice sites are responsible for the *rev* dependence of env mRNA. J Virol 1994; 68:2986-2993.

329. Malim MH, Cullen BR. *Rev* and the fate of pre-mRNA in the nucleus: Implications for the regulation of RNA processing in eukaryotes. Molec Cel Biol 1993; 13:6180-6189.

330. Schwartz S, Felber BK, Pavlakis GN. Distinct RNA sequences in the gag region of human immunodeficiency virus type 1 decrease RNA stability and inhibit expression in the absence of *rev* protein. J Virol 1992; 66:150-159.

331. Maldarelli F, Martin MA, Strebel K. Identification of posttranscriptionally active inhibitory sequences in human immunodeficiency virus type 1 RNA: novel level of gene regulation. J Virol 1991; 65:5732-5743.

332. Cochrane AW, Jones KS, Beidas S, Dillon PJ, Skalka AM, Rosen CA. Identification and characterization of intragenic sequences which repress human immunodeficiency virus structural gene expression. J Virol 1991; 65:5305-5313.

333. D'Agostino D, Felber BK, Harrison JE, Pavlakis GN. The *rev* protein of human immunodeficiency virus type 1 promotes polysomal association and translation of gag/pol and vpu/env mRNAs. Molec Cell Biol 12: 1992; 1375-1386.

334. Lawrence JB, Cochrane AW, Johnson CV, Perkins A, Rosen CA. The HIV-1 *rev* protein: a model system for coupled RNA transport and translation. New Biol 1991; 3:1220-1232.

335. Arrigo S, Chen ISY. *Rev* is necessary for translation but not cytoplasmic accumulation of HIV-1 vif, vpr, and env/vpu 2 mRNAs. Genes Dev 1991; 5:808-819.

336. Malim MH, Cullen BR. HIV-1 structural gene expression requires the binding of multiple *rev* monomers to the viral RRE: Implications for HIV-1 latency. Cell 1991; 65:241-248.

337. Olsen HS, Cochrane AW, Dillon PJ Nalin CM, Rosen CA. Interaction of the human immunodeficiency virus type 1 *rev* protein with a structured region in env mRNAs is dependent on multimer formation mediated through a basic stretch of amino acids. Gene Dev 1990; 4:1357-1364.

338. Zapp ML, Hope TJ, Parslow TG, Green MR. Oligomerization and RNA binding domains of the HIV-1 *rev* protein: a dual function for an arginine-rich bonding motif. Proc Natl Acad Sci USA 1991; 88:7734-7738.

339. Lazinski D, Grzadzielska E, Das A. Sequence-specific recognition of RNA hairpins by bacteriophage antiterminators requires a conserved arginine-rich motif. Cell 1989; 59:207-218.

340. Nalin CM, Purcell RD, Antelman D, Mueller D, Tomchak L, Wegrzynski D, McCarney E, Toome V, Kramer R, Hsu M-C. Purification and characterization of recombinant *rev* protein of human immunodeficiency virus type 1. Proc Natl Acad Sci USA 1990; 87:7593-7597.

341. Heaphy S, Finch JT, Gait MJ, Karn J, Singh M. Human immunodeficiency virus type 1 regulator of viron expression, *rev*, forms nucleoprotein filaments after binding to a purine rich "bubble" located within the *rev*-responsive region of viral RNAs. Proc Natl Acad Sci USA 1991; 88:5704.

342. Hope TJ, Klein NP, Elder ME, Parslow TG. Trans-dominant inhibition of human immunodeficiency virus type 1 *rev* occurs through formation of inactive protein complexes. J Virol 1992; 66:1849-1855.

343. Kjems J, Calnan BJ, Frankel AD, Sharp PA. Specific binding of a basic peptide from HIV-1 *rev*. EMBO J 1992; 11:1119-1129.

344. Iwai S, Pritchard C, Mann DA, Karn J, Gait MJ. Recognition of the high affinity binding site in *rev*-response element RNA by the human immunodeficiency virus type 1 *rev* protein. Nucl Acid Res 1992; 20:6465-6472.

345. Daly TJ, Rennert P, Lynch,P, Barry JK, Dundas M, Rusche JR, Doten RC, Auer M, Farrington GK. Perturbation of the carboxy terminus of HIV-1 *rev* affects multimerization on the *rev* responsive element. Biochem 1993; 32:8945-8954.

346. Perkins A, Cochrane AW, Ruben SM, Rosen CA. Structural and functional characterization of the human immunodeficiency virus type 1 *rev* protein. J AIDS 1989; 2:256-263.

347. Venkatesh LK, Mohammed S, Chinnadurai G. Functional domains of the HIV-1 *rev* gene required for trans-regulation and subcellular localization. Virology 1990; 176:39-47.

348. Hope TJ, McDonald D, Huang XJ, Low J, Parslow TG. Mutational analysis of the human immunodeficiency virus type 1 *rev* transactivator: essential residues near the amino terminus. J Virol 1990; 64:5360-5366.

349. Olsen HS, Beidas S, Dillon P, Rosen CA, Cochrane AW. Mutational analysis of the HIV-1 *rev* protein and its target sequence, the *rev* response element. J AIDS 1991; 4:558-567.

350. Malim MH, Bohnlein S, Hauber J, Cullen BR. Functional dissection of the HIV-1 *rev* trans-activator—derivation of a trans-dominant repressor of *rev* function. Cell 1989; 58:205-214.

351. McDonald D, Hope TJ, Parslow TG. Post-transcriptional regulation by the human immunodeficiency virus type 1 *rev* and human T-cell leukemia virus type 1 *rex* proteins through a heterologous RNA binding site. J

Virol 1992; 66:7232-7238.

352. Malim MH, McCarn DF, Tiley LS, Cullen BR. Mutational definition of the human immunodeficiency virus type 1 *rev* activation domain. J Virol 1991; 65:4248-4254.

353. Malim MH, Bohnlein S, Fenrick R, Le S-Y, Maixel JV, Cullen BR. Functional comparison of the *rev* trans-activators encoded by different primate immunodeficiency virus species. Proc Nat Acad Sci USA 1989; 86:8222-8226.

354. Weichselbraun I, Farrington GK, Rusche JR, Bohnlein E, Hauber J. Definition of the human immunodeficiency virus type 1 *rev* and human T-cell leukemia virus type 1 *rex* protein activation domain by functional exchange. J Virol 1992; 66:2583-2587.

355. Venkatesh LK, Chinnadurai G. Mutants in a conserved region near the carboxy-terminus of HIV-1 *rev* identify functionally important residues and exhibit a dominant negative phenotype. Virology 1990; 178:327-330.

356. Bohnlein S, Pirker FP, Hofer L, Zimmermann K, Bachmayer H, Bohnlein E, Hauber J. Transdominant repressors for human T-cell leukemia virus type 1 and human immunodeficiency virus type 1 *rev* function. J Virol 1991; 65:81-88.

357. Mermer B, Felber BK, Campbell M, Pavlakis GN. Identification of transdominant HIV-1 *rev* protein mutants by direct transfer of bacterially produced proteins into human cells. Nucleic Acid Res 1990; 18:2037-2044.

358. Hope TJ, Bond BL, McDonald D, Klein NP, Parslow TG. Effector domain of human immunodeficiency virus type 1 *rev* and human T-cell leukemia virus type I *rex* are functionally interchangeable and are an essential peptide motif. J Virol 1991; 65:6001-6007.

359. Tiley LS, Malim MH, Cullen BR. Conserved functional organization of the human immunodeficiency virus type and visna virus *rev* proteins. J Virol 1991; 65:3877-3881.

360. Garrett ED, Cullen BR. Comparative analysis of *rev* function in human immunodeficiency viruses type 1 and 2. J Virol 1992; 66:4288-4294.

361. Trono D, Baltimore D. A human cell factor is essential for HIV-1 *rev* action. EMBO J 1990; 9:4155-4160.

362. Ahmed YF, Hanly SM, Malim MH, Cullen BR, Greene WC. Structure-function analyses of the HTLV-1 *rex* and HIV-1 *rev* RNA response elements: insights into the mechanism of *rex* and *rev* action. Genes Dev 1990; 4:1014-1022.

363. Fankhauser C Izaurralde E, Adachi Y, Wingfield P, Laemmli UK. Specific complex of human immunodeficiency virus type 1 *rev* and nucleolar B23 proteins: dissociation by the *rev* response element. Molec Cell Biol 1991; 11:2567-2575.

364. Borer RA, Lehner CF, Eppenberger HM, Nigg EA. Major nucleolar proteins shuttle between nucleus and cytoplasm. Cell 1989; 56:379-390.

365. Vaishnav YN, Vaishnav M, Wong-Staal F. Identification and characterization of a nuclear factor that specifically binds to the *rev*-response element (RRE) of human immunodeficiency virus type 1 (HIV-1). New Biol 1991; 3:142-150.

366. Shulka RR, Kimmel PL, Kumar A. Human immunodeficiency virus type 1 *rev*-responsive element RNA binds to host cell-specific proteins. J Virol 1994; 68:2224-2229.

367. Kjems J, Frankel AD, Sharp PA. Specific regulation of mRNA splicing in vitro by a peptide from HIV-1. Rev Cell 1991; 67:169-178.

368. Kjems J, Sharp PA. The basic domain of *rev* from human immunodeficiency virus type 1 specifically blocks the entry ofU4/U6*U5 small nuclear ribonucleoprotein in spliceosome assembly. J Virol 1993; 67:4769-4776.

369. Ruhl M, Himmelspach M, Bahr GM, Hammerschmid F, Jaksche H, Wolff B, Aschauer H, Farrington GK, Probst H, Bevec D, Hauber J. Eukaryotic initiation factor 5A is a cellular target of the human immunodeficiency virus type 1 *rev* activation domain mediating trans-activation. J Cell Biol 1993; 123:1309-1320.

370. Kim S, Byrn R, Groopman J, Baltimore D. Temporal aspects of DNA and RNA synthesis during human immunodeficiency virus infection: evidence for differential gene expression. J Virol 1989; 63:3708-3713.

371. Dayton ET, Konings DAM, Lim SY, Hsu RKS, Butini L, Pantaleo G, Dayton AI. The RRE of human immunodeficiency virus type 1 contributes to cell-type-specific viral tropism. J Virol 1993; 67:2871-2878.

372. Duan L, Bagasra O, Laughlin MA, Oakes JW, Pomerantz RJ. Potent inhibition of human immunodeficiency virus type 1 replication by an intracellular anti-*rev* single chain antibody. Proc Natl Acad Sci USA 1994; 91: 5075-5079.

373. Selby MJ, Bain ES, Luciw PA, Peterlin BM. Structure, sequence, and position of the stem-loop in tar determine transcriptional elongation by *tat* through the HIV-1 long terminal repeat. Genes Dev 1989; 3:547-558.

374. Graeble MA, Churcher MJ, Lowe AD et al. Human immunodeficiency virus type 1 transactivator protein, *tat*, stimulates transcriptional readthrough of distal terminator sequences in vitro. Proc Natl Acad Sci USA 1993; 90:6184-6188.

375. Feinberg MB, Baltimore D, Frankel AD. The role of *tat* in the human immunodeficiency virus life cycle indicates a primary effect on transcriptional elongation. Proc Natl Acad Sci USA 1991; 88:4045-4049.

376. Saksela K, Stevens C, Rubinstein P, Baltimore D. HIV-1 mRNA expression in PBMC predicts disease progression independent of the numbers of CD4+ lymphocytes. Proc Natl Acad Sci USA 1994; 91: 1104-1108.

377. Malim MH, Hauber J, Fenrick R, Cullen BR. Immunodeficiency virus *rev* trans-activator modulates the expression of the viral regulatory genes. Nature 1988; 335:181-183.

378. Pomerantz RJ, Trono D, Feinberg MB, Baltimore D. Cells nonproductively infected with HIV-1 exhibit an aberrant pattern of viral RNA expression: a molecular model for latency. Cell 1990; 61:1271-1276.

379. Michael NL, Morrow P, Mosca J et al. Induction of human immunodeficiency virus type 1 expression in chronically infected cells is associated primarily with a shift in RNA splicing patterns. J Virol 1991; 65:1291-1303.

379a. Michael NL, Vahey M, Burke DS, Redfield RR. Viral DNA and mRNA expression correlate with the stage of HIV-1 infection in humans: Evidence for viral replication at all stages of HIV disease. J Virol 1992; 66: 310-316.

380. Seshamma T, Bagasra O, Trono D et al. Blocked early stage latency in the peripheral blood cells of certain individuals infected with human im-

munodeficiency virus type 1. Proc Natl Acad Sci USA 1992; 89:10663-10667.

381. Verdin E, Becker N, Bex F et al. Identification and characterization of an enhancer in the coding region of the genome of human immunodeficiency virus type 1. Proc Natl Acad Sci USA 1990; 87:4874-4878.

382. Van Lint C, Burny A, Verdin E. The intragenic enhancer of human immunodeficiency virus type 1 contains functional AP-1 binding sites. J Virol 1991; 65:7066-7072.

383. Verdin E. DNase I-hypersensitive sites are associated with both long terminal repeats and with the intragenic enhancer of integrated human immunodeficiency virus type 1. J Virol 1991; 65:6790-6799.

384. Garcia JA, Wu FK, Mitsuyasu R, Gaynor RB. Interactions of cellular proteins involved in the transcriptional regulation of the human immunodeficiency virus. EMBO J 1987; 6:3761-3770.

385. Desai-Yajnik V, Samuels H. The NF-κB and Sp-1 motifs of the human immunodeficiency virus type 1 long terminal repeat functions as novel thyroid hormone response elements. Molec Cell Biol 1993; 13:5057-5069.

386. Jones KA, Kadonga JT, Luciw PA et al. Activation of the AIDS retrovirusa promoter by the cellular transcription factor Sp-1. Science 1986; 232:755-759.

387. Harrich D, Garcia J, Wu F et al. Role of Sp-1 binding domains in in vivo transcriptional regulation of the human immunodeficiency virus type 1 long terminal repeat. J Virol 1989; 63:2585-2591.

388. Parrot C, Seidner T, Duh E et al. Variable role of the long terminal repeat Sp-1-binding sites in human immunodeficiency virus replication in T-lymphocytes. J Virol 1991; 65:1414-1419.

389. Ross EK, Buckler-White AJ, Robson AB et al. Contribution of NF-κB and Sp-1 binding motifs to the replicative capacity of human immunodeficiency virus type 1: distinct patterns of viral growth are determined by T-cell types. J Virol 1991; 65:4350-4358.

390. Kim JYH, Gonzalez-Scarano F, Zeichner SL et al. Replication of type 1 human immunodeficiency viruses containing linker substitution mutations in the -201 to -130 region of the long terminal repeat. J Virol 1993; 67:1658-1662.

391. Okamoto T, Benter T, Josephs SF, Sadaie MR, Wong-Staal F. Transcriptional activation from the long terminal repeat of human immunodeficiency virus in vitro. Virology 1990; 177:606-614.

392. Sakaguchi M, Zenzie-Gregory B, Groopman JE, Smale S, Kim S Alternative pathway for induction of human immunodeficiency virus gene expression: involvement of the general transcription machinery. J Virol 1991; 65:5448-5456.

393. Gaynor R. Cellular transcription factors involved in the regulation of HIV-1 gene expression. AIDS 1992; 6:347-363.

394. Courey AJ, Tjian R. Analysis of Sp-1 in vivo reveals multiple transcriptional domains including a novel glutamine-rich activation motif. Cell 1989; 55:887-898.

395. Pascal E, Tjian R. Different activation domains of Sp-1 govern formation of multimers and mediate transcriptional synergism. Genes Dev 1991; 5:1646-1656.

396. Mastrangelo IA, Courey AJ, Wall JS, Jackson SP, Hough PVC. DNA

looping and Sp-1 multimer links: a mechanism for transcriptional synergism and enhancement. Proc natl Acad Sci USA 1991; 88:5670-5674.

397. Imataka H, Sogawa K, Yasumoto K, Kikuchi Y, Sasano K, Kobayashi A,
Hayami M, Fujii-Kuriyama Y. Two regulatory proteins that bind to the
basic transcription element (BTE), a GC box sequence in the promoter
region of the rat P-4501A1 gene. EMBO J 1992; 11:3663-3671.

398. Jackson SP, MacDonald J, Lees-Miller S. GC box binding induces phosphorylation of Sp-1 by a DNA-dependent protein kinase Cell 1990;
63:155-165.

399. Su W, Jackson S, Tjian R, Echols H. DNA looping between sites for
transcriptional activation: self-association of DNA-bound Sp-1. Genes Dev
1991; 5:820-826.

400. Perkins ND, Edwards NL, Duckett CS, Agranoff AB, Schmid RM, Nabel
GJ. A cooperative interaction between NF-κB and Sp-1 is required for
HIV-1 enhancer activation EMBO J 1993; 12:3551-3558.

401. Razin A, Cedar H. DNA methylation and gene expression. Microbiol Rev
1991; 55:451-458.

402. Doerfler W. DNA methylation and gene activity. Annu Rev Biochem
1983; 52:93-124.

403. Bednarik DP, Cook AJ, Pitha PM. Inactivation of the HIV LTR by DNA
CpG methylation: evidence for a role in latency. EMBO J 1990; 9:1157-
1164.

404. Bednarik DP, Mosca JD, Raj NBK. Methylation as a modulator of expression of the human immunodeficiency virus. J Virol 1987; 61:1253-
1257.

405. Gutekunst KA, Kashanchi F, Brady JN, Bednarik DP. Transcription of
the HIV-1 LTR is regulated by the density of DNA CpG methylation. J
AIDS 1993; 6:541-549.

406. Boyes J, Bird A. DNA methylation inhibits transcription indirectly via a
methyl-CpG binding protein. Cell 1991; 64:1123-1134.

407. Boyes J, Bird A. Repression of genes by DNA methylation depends on
CpG density and promoter strength: evidence for involvement of a methyl-CpG binding protein. EMBO J 1992; 11:327-333.

408. Lewis JD, Meehan RR, Henzel WJ, Maurer-Fogy I, Jeppesen P, Klein F,
Bird A. Purification, sequence, and cellular localization of a novel chromosomal protein that binds to methylated DNA. Cell 1992; 69:905-914.

409. Meehan RR, Lewis JD, McKay S, Kleiner EL, Bird AP. Identification of
a mammalian protein that binds to methylated DNA. Cell 1989; 58:499-
507.

410. Joel P, Shao W, Pratt K. A nuclear protein with enhanced binding to
methylated Sp-1 sites in the AIDS virus promoter. Nucl Acid Res 1993;
21:5786-5793.

411. Bednarik DP, Duckett C, Kim SU, Perez VL, Griffis K, Guenthner PC,
Folks TM. DNA CpG methylation inhibits binding of NF-κB proteins
to the HIV-1 long terminal repeat cognate DNA motifs. New Biol 1991;
3:969-976.

412. Imataka H, Mizuno A, Fujii-Kuriyama Y, Hayami M. Activation of the
human immunodeficiency virus type 1 long terminal repeat by BTEB a
GC box-binding transcription factor. AIDS Res and Human Retrov 1993;
9:825-831.

413. Dynlacht BD, Hoey T, Tjian R. Isolation of coactivators associated with the TATA-binding protein that mediate transcriptional activation. Cell 1991; 66:563-576.

414. Meisterernst Mand Roeder RG. Family of proteins that interact with TFIID and regulate promoter activity. Cell 1991; 67:557-567.

415. Pugh BF, Tjian R. Diverse transcriptional functions of the multisubunit eukaryotic TFIID complexes. J Biol Chem 1992; 267:679-682.;

416. Tjian R, Maniatis T. Transcriptional activation: A complex puzzle with few easy pieces. Cell 1994; 77:5-8,

417. Burakowski S. The basics of basal transcription by RNA polymerase II. Cell 1994; 77:1-3.

418. Nakajima N, Horikoshi M, Roeder RG. Factors involved in specific transcription by mammalian RNA polymerase II: purification, genetic specificity and TATA box-promoter interactions of TFIID. Molec Cell Biol 1988; 8:4028-4040.

419. Buratowski S, Hahn S, Guerente L et al. Five intermediate complexes in transcription interaction by RNA polymerase II. Cell 198956:549-561.

420. Conaway RC, Conaway JW. General initiation factors for RNA polymerase II. Annu Rev Biochem 1993; 62:161-190.

421. Zawel L, Reinberg D. Initiation of transcription by RNA polymerase II: a multi-step process. Prog Nucl Acids Res Molec Biol 1993; 44:67-108.

422. Kretzschmar M, Kaiser K, Lottspeich F, Meisterernst M. A novel mediator of class II gene transcription with homology to viral immediate-early transcriptional regulators. Cell 1994; 78:525-534.

423. Ge H, Roeder RG. Purification, cloning, and characterization of a human coactivator, PC4, that mediates transcriptional activation of class II genes. Cell 1994; 78:513-523.

424. Jones KA, Luciw PA, Duchange N. Structural arrangements of the transcription control domains within the 5'-untranslated leader regions of the HIV-1 and HIV-2 promoters. Genes Develop 1988; 2:1101-1114,

425. Meisterernst M, Roy, AL, Lieu HM et al. Activation of class KK gene transcription by regulatory factors in potentiated by a novel activity. Cell 1991; 66:981-993.

426. Duan L, Ozaki I, Oakes JW, Taylor JP, Khalili K, Pomerantz RJ. The tumor suppressor protein p53 strongly alters human immunodeficiency virus type 1 replication. J Virol 1994; 68:4302-4313.

427. Subler MA, martin DW, Deb S. Activation of the human immunodeficiency virus long terminal repeat by transforming mutants of human p53. J Virol 1994; 68:103-110.

428. Kashanchi F, Shibata R, Ross EK, Brady JN, Martin MA. Second-site long terminal repeat (LTR) revertants of replication-defective human immunodeficiency virus: effects of revertant TATA box motifs on virus infectivity, LTR-directed expression, in vitro RNA synthesis, and binding of basal transcription factors TFIId and TFIIA. J Virol 1994; 68:3298-3307.

429. Seto E, Shi Y, Shenk T. YY1 is an initiator sequence-binding protein that directs and activates transcription in vitro. Nature 1991; 354:241-245.

430. Smale ST, Baltimore D. The 'initiator' as a transcription control element. Cell 1989; 57:103-113.

431. Roy AL, Meisterernst M, Pognonec P, Roeder RG. Cooperative interac-

tion of an initiator-binding transcription initiation factor and the helix-loop-helix activator USF. Nature 1991; 354:245-248.

432. Shi Y, Seto E, Chang L-S, Shenk T. Transcriptional repression by YY1 a human GLI-Kruppel-related protein and relief of repression by adenovirus E1A protein. Cell 1991; 67:377-388.

433. Lee J-S, Galvin KM, Shi Y. Evidence for physical interaction between the zinc-finger transcription factors YY1 and Sp-1. Proc Natl Acad Sci USA 1993; 90:6145-6149.

434. Margolis DM, Somasundaran M, Green MR. Human transcription factor YY1 represses human immunodeficiency virus type 1 transcription and virion production. J Virol 1994; 68:905-910.

435. Pierce JW, Lenardo M, Baltimore D. Oligonucleotide that binds nuclear factor NF-κB acts as a lymphoid-specific and inducible enhancer element. Proc Natl Acad Sci USA 1988; 85:1482-1486.

436. Nabel G, Baltimore D. An inducible transcription factor activates expression of human immunodeficiency virus in T cells. Nature 1987; 326:711-713.

437. Kawakami K, Scheidereit C, Roeder RG. Identification and purification of a human immunoglobulin enhancer-binding protein (NF-κB) that activates transcription from a human immunodeficiency virus type 1 promoter in vitro. Proc Natl Acad Sci USA 1988; 85:4700-4704.

438. Sen R, Baltimore D. Multiple nuclear factors interact with the immunoglobulin enhancer sequences. Cell 1986; 46:705-716.

439. Rice NR, Ernst MK In vivo control of NF-κB activation by I-κB. EMBO J 1993; 12:4685-4695.

440. Baeuerle PA, Baltimore D. Activation of DNA-binding activity in an apparently cytoplasmic precursor of the NF-κB transcription factor. Cell 1988; 53:211-217.

441. Kieran M, Blank V, Logeat J et al. The DNA binding subunit of NF-κB is identical to factor KBF-1 and homologous to the rel oncogene product. Cell 1990; 62:1007-1018.

442. Liou H-C, Baltimore D. Regulation of the NF-κB/rel transcription factor and I-κB inhibitor system. Curr Opin Cell Biol 1993; 5:477-487.

443. Molitor JA, Walker WH, Doerre S et al. NF-κB: a family of inducible and differentially expressed enhancer binding proteins in human T-cells. Proc Nat Acad Sci USA 1990; 87:10028-10032.

444. Lenardo MJ, Baltimore D. NF-κB: A pleiotropic mediator of inducible and tissue specific gene control. Cell 1989; 58:227-229.

445. Schmid RM, Perkins ND, Duckett CS et al. Cloning of an NF-κB subunit which stimulates HIV transcription in synergy with p65. Nature 1991; 352:733-736.

446. Mercurio F, DiDonato JA, Rosette C, Karin M. p105 and p98 precursor proteins play an active role in NF-κB-mediated signal transduction. Genes Dev 1993; 7:705-717.

447. Riviere Y, Blank V, Kourilsky P, Israel A. Processing of the precursor of NF-κB by the HIV-1 protease during acute infection. Nature 1991; 350:625-626.

448. Fan C-M, Maniatis T. Generation of p50 subunit of NF-κB by processing of p105 through an ATP-dependent pathway. Nature 1991; 354:395-398.

449. Blank V, Kourilsky P, Israel A. Cytoplasmic retention, DNA binding and processing of the NF-κB p50 precursor are controlled by a small region in its C-terminus. EMBO J 1991; 10:4159-4167.

450. Fujita T, Nolan GP, Ghosh S, Baltimore D. Independent modes of transcriptional activation by the p50 and p65 subunits of NF-κB. Genes Dev 1992; 6:775-787.

451. Baeuerle PA, Baltimore D. A 65-kD subunit of active NF-κB is required for inhibition of NF-κB by I-κB. Genes Dev 1989; 3:1689-1698.

452. Kieran M, Blank V, Logeat F, Vandekerckhove J, Lottspeich F, Bail OL, Urban MB, Kourilsky P, Baeuerle PA, Israel A. The DNA binding subunit of NF-κB is identical to factor KBF1 and homologous to the rel oncogene product. Cell 1990; 62:1007-1018.

453. Nolan GP, Ghosh S, Liou H-C et al. DNA binding and I-κB inhibition of the cloned p65 subunit of NF-κB a rel-related polypeptide. Cell 1991; 64:961-969.

454. Logeat F, Israel N, Ten R et al. Inhibition of transcription factors belonging to the rel/NF-κB family by a transdominant negative mutant. EMBO J 1991; 10:1827-1832.

455. Ruben SM, Dillon PJ, Schereck R et al. Isolation of a rel-related human cDNA that potentially encodes the 65-kD subunit of NF-κB. Science 1991; 251:1490-1493.

456. Rattner A, Korner M, Rosen PA et al. Nuclear factor κB activates proencephalin transcription in T lymphocytes. Molec Cell Biol 1991; 11:1017-1022.

457. Kretzschmar M, Meisterernst M, Scheidereit C et al. Transcriptional regulation of the HIV-1 promoter by NF-κB in vitro. Gene Dev 1992; 6:761-774.

458. Schmitz ML, Baeuerle PA. The p65 subunit is responsible for the strong transcription activating potential of NF-κB. EMBO J 1991; 10:3805-3817.

459. Franzoso G, Bours V, Azarenko V et al. The oncoprotein Bcl-3 can facilitate NF-κB mediated transactivation by removing inhibiting p50 homodimers from select κB sites. EMBO J 1993; 12:3893-3901.

460. Franzoso G, Bours V, Park S et al. The candidate oncoprotein Bcl-3 is an antagonist of p50/NF-κB-mediated inhibition. Nature 1992; 359:339-342.

461. Kang S-M, Tran A, Grilli M et al. NF-κB subunit regulation in non-transformed CD4+ T-lymphocytes. Science 1992; 256:1452-1456.

462. Doerre S, Sista P, Sun S-C et al. The c-rel protooncogene product represses NF-κB p65 mediated transcriptional activation of the long terminal repeat of type 1 human immunodeficiency virus. Proc Natl Acad Sci USA 1993; 90:1023-1027.

463. Bours V, Burd PR, Brown K et al. A novel mitogen-inducible gene product related to p50/p105-NF-κB participates in transactivation through a κB site. Molec Cell Biol 1992; 12:685-695.

464. Neri A, Chang C-C, Lombardi L et al. B cell lymphoma-associated chromosomal translocation involves andidate oncogene, lyt-10, homologuus to NF-κB p50. Cell 1991; 67:1075-1087.

465. Haskill S, Beg AA, Tompkins SM et al. Characterization of an immediate-early gene induced in adherent monocytes that encodes I-κB-like activity. Cell 1991; 65:1281-1289.

466. Davis N, Ghosh S, Simmons DL et al. Rel-associated pp40: an inhibitor of the rel family of transcription factors. Science 1991; 253:1268-1271.

467. Liou H-C, Nolan GP, Ghosh S et al. The NF-κB p50 precursor, p105, contains an internal I-kB-like inhibitor that preferentially inhibits p50. EMBO J 1992; 11:3003-3009.

468. Inoue J-I, Kerr LD,Kakizuka A et al. I-κB a 70kD protein identical to the C-terminal half of p110 NF-κB: a new member of the I-κB family. Cell 1992; 68:1109-1120.

469. Hatada EN, Nieters A, Wulczyn FG et al. The ankyrin repeat domain of the NF-κB precursor p105 and the proto-oncogene blc-3 act as specific inhibitors of NF-κB DNA binding. Proc Natl Acad Sci USA 1992; 89:2489-2493.

470. Henkel T, Machleidt T, Alkalay I et al. Rapid proteolysis of I-κB-α is necessary for activation of transcription factor NF-κB. Nature 1993; 365:182-184.

471. Ten RM, Paya CV, Israel N et al. The characterization of the promoter of the gene encoding the p50 subunit of NF-κB indicates that it participates in its own regulation. EMBO J 1992; 11:195-203.

472. Bagasra O, Wright SD, Seshamma T et al. CD14 is involved in control of human immunodeficiency virus type 1 expression in latently infected cells by lipopolysaccharide. Proc Natl Acad Sci USA 1992; 89:6285-6289.

473. Dinter H, Chiu R, Imagawa M et al. In vitro activation of the HIV-1 enhancer in extracts from cells treated with a phorbol ester tumor promoter. EMBO J 1987; 6:4067-4071.

474. Kaufman JD, Valandra G, Roderiquez G et al. Phorbol ester enhances human immunodeficiency virus-promoted gene expression and acts on a repeated 10 base pair functional enhancer element. Molec Cell Biol 1987; 7:3759-3766.

475. Bours V, Villalobos J, Burd PR et al. Cloning of a mitogen inducible gene encoding a κB DNA binding protein with homology to the rel oncogene and to cell cycle motifs. Nature 1990; 348:76-79.

476. Legrand-Poels S, Vaira D, Pincemail J et al. Activation of human immunodeficiency virus type 1 by oxidative stress. AIDS Res Human Retrov. 1990; 12:1389-1397.

477. Schreck R, Rieber P, Baeuerle PA. Reactive oxygen intermediates as apparently widely used messengers in the activation of the NF-κB transcription factor and HIV-1 EMBO J 1991; 10:2247-2258.

478. Osborn L, Kunkel S, Nabel GJ. Tumor necrosis factor α and interleukin 1 stimulate the human immunodeficiency virus enhancer by activation of the nuclear factor κB. Proc Natl Acad Sci USA 1989; 86:2336-2340.

479. Broor S, Kusari AB, Zhang B et al. Stimulation of HIV replication in mononuclear phagocytes by leukemia inhibitory factor. J AIDS 1994; 7:647-654.

480. Arenzana-Seisdedos F, Fernandez B, Dominguez I et al. Phosphatidylcholine hydrolysis activates NF-κB and increases human immunodeficiency virus replication in human monocytes and T lymphocytes. J Virol 1993; 67:6596-6604.

481. Quinto I, Ruocco MR, Baldassarre F et al. The human immunodeficiency virus type 1 long terminal repeat is activated by monofunctional and bifunctional alkylating agents in human lymphocytes. J Biol Chem 1993;

268:26719-26724.

482. Ostrove JM, Leonard J, Weck KE et al. Activation of the human immunodeficiency virus by herpes simplex virus type 1. J Virol 1987; 61:3726-3732.

483. Peterson PK, Gekker G, Chao CC et al. Human cytomegalovirus stimulated peripheral blood mononuclear cells induce HIV-1 replication via a tumor necrosis α mediated mechanism. J Clin Invest 1992; 89:574-580.

484. Scala G, Quinto I, Ruocco MR et al. Epstein-Barr virus nuclear antigen 2 transactivates the long terminal repeat of human immunodeficiency virus type 1. J Virol 1993; 67:2853-2861.

485. Leonard J, Parrott C, Buckler-White AJ et al. The NF-κB binding sites in the human immunodeficiency virus type 1 long terminal repeat are not required for virus infectivity. J Virol 1989; 63:4919-4924.

486. Lu Y, Touzjian N, Stenzel M, Dorfman T, Sodroski JG, Haseltine WA. The NF-κB independent cis-acting sequences in HIV-1 LTR responsive to T-cell activation. J AIDS 1991; 4:173-177.

487. Lu Y, Stenzel M, Sodroski JG et al. Effects of long terminal repeat mutations on human immunodeficiency virus type 1 replication. J Virol 1989; 63:4115-4119.

488. Rosen CA, Sodroski JG, Haseltine WA. The location of Cis acting regulatory sequences in the human T cell lymphotropic virus type III (HTLV-III/LAV) long terminal repeat. Cell 1985; 41:813-823.

489. Siekevitz M, Josephs SF, Dukovich M et al. Activation of the HIV-1 LTR by T cell mitogens and the trans-activator protein of HTLV-1. Science 1987; 238:1575-1578.

490. Zeichner SL, Kim JYH, Alwine JC. Linker scanning mutational analysis of the transcriptional activity of the human immunodeficiency virus type 1 long terminal repeat. J Virol 1991; 65:2436-2444.

491. Lenardo MJ, Fan C-M, Maniatis T, Baltimore D. The involvement of NF-κB in β-interferon gene regulation reveals its role as widely inducible mediator of signal transduction. Cell 1989; 57:287-294.

492. Ron D, Brasier AR, Habener JF. Angiotensinogen gene-inducible enhancer binding protein 1 a member of a new family of large nuclear proteins that recognize nuclear factor κB binding sites through a zinc finger motif. Molec Cell Biol 1991; 11:2887-2895.

493. Whelan J, P. Ghersa RH van Huijsduijnen et al. An NF-κB-like factor is essential but not sufficient for cytokine induction of endothelial leukocyte adhesion molecule 1 (ELAM-1) gene transcription. Nucl Acid Res 1991; 19:2645-2653.

494. Brown AM, Linhoff MW, Stein B et al. Function of NF-κB/Rel binding sites in the major histocompatibility complex class II invariant chain promoter is dependent on cell-specific binding of different NF-κB/Rel subunits. Molec Cell Biol 1994; 14:2926-2935.

495. Hansen SK, Nerlov C, Zabel U et al. A novel complex between the p65 subunit of NF-κB and c-Rel binds to a DNA element involved in the phorbol ester induction of the human urokinase gene. EMBO J 1992; 11:205-213.

496. Franza Jr BR, Josephs SF, Gilman MZ et al. Characterization of cellular proteins recognizing the HIV enhancer using a microscale DNA affinity precipitation assay. Nature 1987; 330:391-395.

497. Wu FK, Garcia JA, Harrich D, Gaynor RB. Purification of the human immunodeficiency virus type 1 enhancer and TAR binding proteins EBP-1 and UBP-1. EMBO J 1988; 7:2117-2129.

498. Baldwin AS, Sharp PA. Two transcription factors, NF-κB and H2TF1, interact with a single regulatory sequence in the class I major histocompatibility complex promoter. Proc Natl Acad Sci USA 1988; 85:723-727.

499. Macchi M, Bornert JM, Davidson I et al. THe SV 40 TCII (κB) enhancer binds ubiquitous and cell type specific inducible muclear proteins from lymphoid and non-lymphoid cell lines. EMBO J 1989; 8:4215-4227.

500. Fan CM, Maniatis T. A DNA-binding protein containing two widely separated zinc finger motifs that recognize the same DNA sequence. Gene Dev 1990; 4:29-42.

501. Muchardt C, Seeler JS, Nirula A et al. Regulation of human immunodeficiency virus enhancer function by PRDII-BF1. J Virol 1992; 66:244-250.

502. Baldwin AS, LeClair KP, Harinder S et al. A large protein containing zinc finger domains binds to related sequence elements in the enhancers of the class I major histocompatibility complex and kappa immunoglobulin genes. Molec Cell Biol 1990; 10:1406-1414.

503. Seeler J-S, Muchardt C, Suessle A et al. Transcription factor PRDII-BF1 activates human immunodeficiency virus type 1 gene expression. J Virol 1994; 68:1002-1009.

504. Seth A, Ascione R, Fisher RJ et al. The ets gene family. Cell Growth Differ 1992; 3:327-334.

505. Holzmeister J, Ludewig B, Pauli G et al. Sequence specific binding of the transcription factor c-ets1 to the human immunodeficiency virus type 1 long terminal repeat. Biochem Biophys Res Comm 1993; 3:1229-1233.

506. Bousselut R, Duvall JF, Gegonne A et al. The product of the c-ets-1 proto-oncogene and the related Ets2 protein act as transcriptional activators of the long terminal repeat of human T cell leukemia virus HTLV-1. EMBO J 1990; 9:3137-3144.

507. Gunther CV, Nye JA, Bryner RS et al. Sequence specific DNA binding of the proto-oncogene ets-1 defines a transcriptional activator sequence within the long terminal repeat of the Moloney murine sarcoma virus. Gene Dev 1990; 4:667-679.

508. Seth A, Hodge DR, Thompson DM et al. ETS family proteins activate transcription from HIV-1 long terminal repeat. AIDS Res Hum Retrov 1993; 10:1017-1023.

509. Jones KA. HIV trans-activation and transcription control mechanism. New Biol 1989; 1:127-135.

510. Lu Y, Touzjian N, Stenzel M et al. Identification of cis-acting repressive sequences within the negative regulatory element of human immunodeficiency virus type 1. J Virol 1990; 64:5226-5229.

511. Franza Jr BR, Rauscher III FJ Josephs SF et al. The fos complex and fos-related antigens recognize sequence elements that contain AP-1 binding sites. Science 1988; 239:1150-1153.

512. Shaw JP, Utz PJ, Durand DB et al. Identification of a putative regulator of early T cell activation genes. Science 1988; 241:202-205.

513. Li C, Lai C, Sigman DS, Gaynor RB. Cloning of a cellular factor, interleukin binding factor, that binds to NFAT-like motifs in the human

immunodeficiency virus long terminal repeat. Proc Natl Acad Sci USA 1991; 88: 7739-7743.

514. Giacca M, Gutierrez MI, Menzo S, Fagagna FDD, Falaschi A. A human binding site for transcription factor USF? MLTF mimics the negative regulatory element of human immunodeficiency virus type 1. Virology 1992; 186: 133-147.

515. Gregor, PD, Sawadogo M, Roeder RG The adenovirus major late transcription factor USF is a member of the helix-loop-helix group of regulatory proteins and binds to DNA as a dimer. Gene Dev 1990; 4:1730-1740.

516. Murre C, McCaw P, Baltimore D. A new DNA-binding and dimerization motif in immunoglobulin enhancer binding, daughterless, myoD, and myc proteins. Cell 1989; 56:777-783.

517. Smith MR, Greene WC. The same 50 kilodalton cellular proteins binds to the negatige regulatory elements of the interleukin-2 receptor α-chain gene and the human immunodeficiency virus type 1 long terminal repeat. Proc Natl Acad Sci USA 1989; 86:8526-8530.

518. Kretzner L, Blackwood EM, Eisenman RN. Myc and Max proteins possess distinct transcriptional activities. Nature 1992; 359:426-429.

519. Workman JL, Roeder RG, Kingston RE. An upstream transcription factor, USF (MLTF), facilitates the formation of preinitiation complexes during in vitro chromatin assembly. EMBO J 1990; 9:1299-1308.

520. Demarchi F, D'Agaro P, Falaschi A, Giacca M. In vivo footprinting analysis of constitutive and inducible protein-DNA interactions at the long terminal repeat of human immunodeficiency virus type 1. J Virol 1993; 67:7450-7460.

521. Fedor MJ, Lue NF, Kornberg RD. Statistical positioning of nucleosomes by specific protein-binding to an upstream activating sequence in yeast. J Molec Biol 1988; 204:109-127.

522. Chasman DI, Lue NF, Buchman AR, LaPointe JW, Lorch Y, Kornberg RD. A yeast protein that influences the chromatin structure of UASG and functions as a powerful auxiliary gene activator. Genes Develop 1990; 4:503-514.

523. Zeichner SL, Kim JYH, Alwine JC. Analysis of the human immunodeficiency virus long terminal repeat by in vitro transcription competition and linker scanning mutagenesis. Gene Expression 1991; 1:15-27.

524. Zeichner SL, Kirka G, Andrews PW, Alwine JC. Differentiation-dependent human immunodeficiency virus long terminal repeat regulatory elements active in human teratocarcinoma cells. J Virol 1992; 66:2268-2273.

525. Tesmer VM, Rajadhyaksha A, Babin J, Bina M. NF-IL6-mediated transcriptional activation of the long terminal repeat of the human immunodeficiency virus type 1. Proc Natl Acad Sci USA 1993; 90:7298-7302.

526. LeClair KP, Blanar MA, Sharp PA. The p50 subunit of NF-κB associates with the NF-IL6 transcription factor. Proc Natl Acad Sci USA 1992; 89:8145-8149.

527. Ray A, Prefontaine KE. Physical association and functional antagonism between the p65 subunit of transcription factor NF-κB and the glucocorticoid receptor. Proc Natl Acad Sci USA 1994; 91:752-756.

529. Orchard K, Lang G, Collins M, Latchman D. Characterization of a novel T-lymphocyte protein which binds to a site related to steroid/thyroid

hormone receptor response elements in the negative regulatory sequence of the human immunodeficiency virus long terminal repeat. Nucl Acid Res 1992; 20:5429-5434.

530. Cooney AJ, Tsai SY, O'Malley BW et al. Chicken ovalbumin upstream promoter transcription factor binds to a negative regulatory region in the human immunodeficiency virus type 1 long terminal repeat. J Virol 1991; 65:2853-2860.

531. Wang LH, Tsai WY, Cook RG et al. COUP transcription factor is a member of the steroid receptor superfamily. Nature 1989; 340:163-166.

532. Waterman ML, Fischer WH, Jones KA. A thymus-specific member of the HMG protein family regulates the human T-cell receptor Cα enhancer. Genes Dev 1991; 5:656-669.

533. Waterman ML, Jones KA. Purification of TCF1α T-cell specific transcription factor that activates the T-cell receptor Cα gene enhancer in a context-dependent manner. New Biol 1990; 2:621-636.

534. Wen L, Huang JK, Johnson BH et al. A human placental cDNA clone that encodes non-histone chromosomal protein HNG-1. Nucl Acid Res 1989; 17:1197-1214.

535. Thanos D, Maniatis T. The high mobility group protein HMG I(Y) is required for NF-κB dependent virus induction of the human IFN-β gene. Cell 1992; 71:777-789.

536. Golub EI, Li G, Volsky DJ. Differences in the basal activation of the long terminal repeat determine different replicative capacities of two closely related human immunodeficiency virus type 1 isolates. J Virol 1990; 64:3654-3660.

537. Jamieson BD, Aldrovanci GM, Planelles V, Jowett JBM, Gao L, Block LM, Chen ISY, Zack JA. Requirement of human immunodeficiency virus type 1 nef for in vivo replication and pathogenicity. J Virol 1994; 68:3478-3485.

538. Kestler HW, Ringler DJ, Mori K, Panicali DL, Sehgal PK, Daniel MD, Desrosiers RC. Importance of the nef gene for maintenance of high virus loads and for development of AIDS. Cell 1991; 65:651-662.

539. Kirchhoff F, Kestler, HW, Desrosiers RC. Upstream U3 sequences in simian immunodeficiency virus are selectively deleted in vivo in the absence of an intact nef gene. J Virol 1994; 68:2031-2037.

540. Malim MH, Fenrick R, Ballard DW et al. Functional characterization of a complex protein-DNA binding domain located within the human immunodeficiency virus type 1 long terminal repeat leader region. J Virol 1989; 63:3213-3219.

541. Kato H, Horikoshi M, Roeder RG. Repression of HIV-1 transcription by a cellular protein. Science 1991; 251:1476-1479.

542. Klaver B, Berkhout B. Comparison of 5' and 3' long terminal repeat promoter function in human immunodeficiency virus. J Virol 1994; 68:3830-3840.

543. Cullen BR, Lomedico PT, Ju G. Transcriptional interference in avian retroviruses—implications for the promoter insertion model of leukaemogenesis. Nature 1984; 307:241-245.

544. Hirschman JE, Durbin KJ, Winston F. Genetic evidence for promoter competition in Saccharomyces cerevisiae. Molec Cell Biol 1988; 8:4608-4615.

545. Ju G, Cullen BR. The role of avian retroviral LTRs in the regulation of gene expression and viral replication. Adv Virus Res 1985; 30: 179-223.

546. Emerman M, Temin HM. Comparison of promoter suppression in avian and murine retrovirus vectors. Nucl Acid Res 1986; 14:9381-9396.

547. Emerman M, Temin HM. Quantitative analysis of gene suppression in integrated retrovirus vectors. Molec Cell Biol 1986; 6:792-800.

548. Emerman M, Temin HM. Genes with promoters in retrovirus vectors can be independently suppressed by an epigenetic mechanism. Cell 1984; 39:459-467.

549. Arrigo S, Yun M, Beemon K. cis-acting elements within the gag genes of avian retroviruses. Molec Cell Biol 1987; 7:388-397.

550. Boerkoel CF, Kung H-J. Transcription interaction between retroviral long terminal repeats (LTRs): mechanism of 5' LTR suppression and 3' LTR promoter activation of c-myc in avian B-cell lymphomas. J Virol 1992; 66:4814-4823.

551. Raineri I, Senn H-P. HIV-1 promoter insertion revealed by selective detection of chimeric provirus-host gene transcripts. Nucl Acid Res 1992; 20:6261-6266.

552. Valsamakis A, Schek N, Alwine JC. Elements upstream of the AAUAAA within the human immunodeficiency virus polyadenylation signal are required for efficient polyadenylation in vitro. Molec Cell Biol 1992; 12:3699-3705.

553. Valsamakis A, Zeichner S, Carswell S et al. The human immunodeficiency virus type 1 polyadenylation signal: a 3' long terminal repeat element upstream of the AAUAAA necessary for efficient polyadenylation. Proc Natl Acad Sci USA 1991; 88:2108-2112.

554. Weichs an der Glon C, Monks J, Proudfoot NJ. Occlusion of the HIV poly(A) site. Genes Dev 1991; 5:244-253.

555. Bohnlein S, Hauber J, Cullen BR. Identification of a U5-specific sequence required for efficient polyadenylation within the human immunodeficiency virus long terminal repeat. J Virol 1989; 63:421-424.

556. Cherrington J, Ganem D. Regulation of polyadenylation in human immunodeficiency virus (HIV): contributions of promoter proximity and upstream sequences. EMBO J 1992; 11:1513-1524.

557. Dezazzo JD, Kilpatrick JE, Imperiale MJ. Involvement of long terminal repeat U3 sequences overlapping the transcription control region in human immunodeficiency virus type 1 mRNA 3'-end formation. Molec Cell Biol 1991; 11:1624-1630.

558. Belec PA, Pratt-Lowe E, Unger RE et al. Cytomegalovirus (CMV) encephalomyeloradiculitis and human immunodeficiency virus (HIV) encephalitis: presence of HIV and CMV co-infected multinucleated giant cells. Acta Neuropathol 1990; 81:381-385.

559. Finkle C, Tapper MA, Knox KK et al. Coinfection of cells with the human immunodeficiency virus and cytomegalovirus in lung tissues of patients with AIDS. J AIDS 1991; 4:735-737.

560. Nelson JA, Reynolds-Kohler C, Oldstone MBA et al. HIV and HCMV coinfect brain cells in patients with AIDS. Virology 1988; 165:286-290.

561. Skolnik PR, Pomerantz RJ, de la Monte SM et al. Dual infection of retina with human immunodeficiency virus type 1 and cytomegalovirus. Am J Ophthalmol 1989; 107:361-372.

562. Barry PA, Pratt-Lowe E, Peterlin BM et al. Cytomegalovirus activates transcription directed by the long terminal repeat of human immunodeficiency virus type 1. J Virol 1990; 64:2932-2940.

563. Biegalke BJ, Geballe AP. Sequence requirements for activation of the HIV-1 LTR by human cytomegalovirus. Virology 1991; 183:381-385.

564. Davis MG, Kenney SC, Kamine J et al. Immediate-early region of human cytomegalovirus trans-activates the promoter of human immunodeficiency virus. Proc Natl Acad Sci USA 1987; 84:8642-8646.

565. Rando RF, Srinivasan A, Feingold J et al. Characterization of multiple molecular interactions between human cytomegalovirus (HCMV) and human immunodeficiency virus type 1 (HIV-1). Virology 1990; 176: 87-97.

566. Stenberg RM, Depto AS, Fortney J et al. Regulated expression of early and late RNAs and proteins for the human cytomegalovirus immediate-early gene region. J Virol 1989; 63:2699-2708.

567. Stinski MF, Thomsen DR, Stenberg RM et al. Organization and expression of the immediate early genes of human cytomegalovirus. J Virol 1983; 49:190-199.

568. Staprans SI, Rabert DK, Spector DH. Identification of sequence requirements and trans-acting functions necessary for regulated expression of a human cytomegalovirus early gene. J Virol 1988; 62:3463-3473.

569. Ghazal P, Young J, Giulietti E et al. A discrete cis element in the human immunodeficiency virus long terminal repeat mediates synergistic trans activation by cytomegalovirus immediate early proteins. J Virol 1991; 65:6735-6742.

570. Klucher KM, Spector DH. The human cytomegalovirus 2.7 kilobase RNA promoter contains a functional binding site for the adenovirus major late transcription factor. J Virol 1990; 64:4189-4198.

571. Markovitz DM, Kenney S, Kamine J et al. Disparate effects of two herpesvirus immediate-early gene trans-activators on the HIV-1 LTR. Virology 1989; 173:750-754.

572. Sambucetti LC, Cherrington JM, Wilkinson GWG et al. NF-κB activation of the cytomegalovirus enhancer is mediated by a viral transactivator and by T cell stimulation. EMBO J 1989; 8:4251-4258.

573. Gaynor RB, Kuwabara MD, Wu FK et al. Repeated B motifs in the human immunodeficiency virus type 1 long terminal repeat enhancer region do not exhibit cooperative factor binding. Proc Natl Acad Sci USA 1988; 85:9406-9410.

574. Hirka G, Prakash K, Kawashima H et al. Differentiation of human embryonal carcinoma cells induces human immunodeficiency virus permissiveness which is stimulated by human cytomegalovirus coinfection. J Virol 1991; 65:2732-2735.

575. Ho W-Z, Harouse JM, Rando RF et al. Reciprocal enhancement of gene expression and viral replication between human cytomegalovirus and human immunodeficiency virus type 1. J Gen Virol 1990; 71:97-103.

576. Ho W-Z, Song L, Douglas SD. Human cytomegalovirus infection and trans-activation of HIV-1 LTR in human brain-derived cells. J AIDS 1990; 4:1098-1106.

577. Koval V, Clark C, Vaishnav SA et al. Human cytomegalovirus inhibits human immunodeficiency virus type 1 replication in cells productively

infected by both viruses. J Virol 1991; 65:6969-6978.

578. Jault FM, Spector SA, Spector DH. The effects of cytomegalovirus on human immunodeficiency virus replication in brain-derived cells correlate with permissiveness of the cell for each virus. J Virol 1994; 68:959-973.

579. Kliewer S, Garcia J, Pearson L et al. Multiple transcriptional regulatory domains in the human immunodeficiency virus type long terminal repeat are involved in basal and E1a/E1B-induced promoter activity. J Virol 1989; 63:4616-4625.

580. Lee WS, Kao CC, Bryant GO et al. Adenovirus E1A activation domain binds the basic repeat in the TATA box transcription factor. Cell 1991; 67:365-376.

581. Mosca JD, Bednarik DP, Raj NBK et al. Herpes simplex virus type 1 can activate transcription of latent human immunodeficiency virus. Nature (London) 1987; 325:67-70.

582. Ostrove JM, Leonard J, Weck KE et al. Activation of the human immunodeficiency virus by herpes simplex virus type 1. J Virol 1987; 61:3726-3732.

583. Mosca JD, Bednarik DP, Raj NBK et al. Activation of human immunodeficiency virus by herpes virus infection: identification of a region within the long terminal repeat that responds to a trans-acting factor encoeded by herpes simplex virus 1. Proc Natl Acad Sci USA 1987; 84:7408-7412.

584. Weber PC, Kenney JJ, Wigdahl B. Antiviral properties of a dominant negative mutant of the herpes simplex virus type 1 regulatory protein ICP0. J Gen Virol 1992; 73:2955-2961.

585. Vlach J, Pitha PM. Differential contribution of herpes simplex virus type 1 gene products and cellular factors to the activation of human immunodeficiency virus type 1 provirus. J Virol 1993; 67:4427-4431.

586. Vlach J, Pitha PM. Herpes simplex virus type 1 mediated induction of human immunodeficiency virus type 1 provirus correlates with binding of nuclear proteins to the NF-κB enhancer and leader sequence. J Virol 1992; 66:3616-3623.

587. Margolis DM, Ostrove JM, Strauss SE. HSV-1 activation of HIV-1 transcription is augmented by a cellular protein that binds near the initiator element. Virology 1993; 192:370-374.

588. Margolis DM, Rabson AB, Straus SE et al. Transactivation of the HIV-1 LTR by HSV-1 immediate-early genes. Virology 1992; 186:788-791.

589. Lusso P, Ensoli B, Markham PD et al. Productive dual infection of human CD4 T lymphocytes by HIV-1 and HHV-6. Nature (London) 1989; 337:370-373.

590. Lusso P, Maris AD, Malnati M et al. Induction of CD4 and susceptibility to HIV-1 infection in human CD8+ T lymphocytes by human herpesvirus 6. Nature (London) 1991; 349:533-535.

591. Levy JA, Landay A, Lennette ET. Human herpes virus 6 inhibits human immunodeficiency virus type 1 replication in cell culture. J Clin Microbiol 1990; 28:2362-2364.

592. Carrigan DR, Knox KK, Tapper MA. Suppression of human immunodeficiency virus type 1 replication by human herpesvirus-6. J Infect Dis 1990; 162:844-851.

593. Ensoli B, Lusso P, Schachter F et al. Human herpesvirus-6 increases HIV-1 expression in co-infected T cells via nuclear factors binding to the HIV-

1 enhancer. EMBO J 1989; 8:3019-3027.

594. Horvat RT, Wood C, Josephs SJ et al. Transactivation of the human immunodeficiency virus promoter by human herpesvirus-6 (HHV-6) strains GS and Z-29 in primary human T lymphocytes and identification of transactivating HHV-6 gene fragments. J Virol 1991; 65:2895-2902.

595. Wang J, Jones C, Norcross M et al. Identification and characterization of a human herpesvirus 6 gene segment capable of transactivating the human immunodeficiency virus type 1 long terminal repeat in an Sp-1 binding site-dependent manner. J Virol 1994; 68:1706-1713.

596. Sabino E, Cheng-Meyer C, Mayer A. An individual with a high prevalence of a *tat*-defective provirus in peripheral blood. AIDS. Res Hum Retrov 1993; 9:1265-1268.

597. Connor RI, Ho DD. Human immunodeficiency virus type 1 variants with increase replicative capacity develop during the asymptomatic stage before disease progression. J Virol 1994; 68:4400-4408.

598. Tersmette M, de Goede REY, Al BJM, Winkel RA, Gruters HT, Huisman HG, Miedema F. Differential syncytium-inducing capacity of human immunodeficiency virus isolates: frequent detection of syncytium-inducing isolates in patients with acquired immunodeficiency syndrome (AIDS) and AIDS-related complex. J Virol 1988; 62:2026-2032.

599. Tersmette M, Gruters R, de Wolf F, de Goede REY, Lange JMA, Schellekens PTA, Goudsmit J, Huisman HG, Meidema F. Evidence for a role of virulent human immunodeficiency virus (HIV) variants in the pathogenesis of acquired immunodeficiency syndrome: studies on sequential isolates. J Virol 1989; 63:2118-2125.

600. Tersmette M, Lange JMA, De Goede REY, de Wolf F, Eefink Schattenkerk JKM, Schellekens PTA, Coutinho RA, Huisman HG, Goudsmith J, Meidema F. Association between biological properties of human immunodeficiency virus variants and risk for AIDS and AIDS mortality. Lancet 1989; i:983-985.

601. Fenyo EM, Morfeldt-Mason L, Chiodi F, Lind B, von Gegerfelt A, Albert J, Olausson E, Asjo B. Distinctive replicative and cytopathic characteristics of human immunodeficiency virus isolates. J Virol 1988; 62:4414-4419.

602. Roos MTL, Lange JMA, de Goede REY, Coutinho RA, Schellenkens PTA, Miedema F, Tersmette M. Viral phenotype and immune response in primary human immunodeficiency virus type infection. J Infect Dis 1992; 165:427-432.

603. Schuitemaker H, Koot M, Koostra A, Dercksen MW, de Goede REY, van Steenwijk RP, Lange JMA, Schattenker JKME, Miedema F, Tersmette M. Biological phenotype of human immunodeficiency virus type 1 clones at different stages of infection: progression of disease is associated with a shift from monocytotropic to T-cell-tropic populations. J Virol 1992; 66:1354-12360.

604. Kornberg RD, Lorch Y. Chromatin structure and transcription. Annu Rev Cell Biol 1992; 8:563-587.

605. Paranjape SM, Kamakaka RT, Kadonaga JT. Role of chromatin structure in the regulation of transcription by RNA polymerase II. Ann Rev Biochem 1994; 63:265-97.

606. Almer A, Horz W. Nuclease hypersensitive regions with adjacent posi-

tioned nucleosomes mark the gene boundaries of the PHO5/PHO3 locus in yeast. EMBO J 1986; 5:2681-2687.

607. Almer A, Rudolph H, Hinnen A et al. Removal of positioned nucleosomes from the yeast PHO5 promoter upon PHO5 induction releases additional upstream activating DNA elements. EMBO J 1986; 5:2689-2696.

608. Ambrose C, Rajadhyaksha A, Lowman H et al. Locations of nucleosomes on the regulatory region of simian virus 40. J Molec Biol 1989; 209: 255-263.

609. Knezetic JA, Jacob GA, Luse DS. Assembly of RNA Polymerase II pre-initiation complexes before assembly of nucleosomes allows efficient initiation of transcription on nucleosomal templates. Molec Cell Biol 1988; 8: 3114-312.

610. Shimamura A, Sapp M, Rodriquez-Campos A et al. Histone 1 represses transcription from mini chromosomes assembled in vitro. Molec Cell Biol 1989; 9:5573-5584.

611. Straka C, Horz W. A functional role for nucleosomes in the repression of a yeast promoter. EMBO J 1991; 10: 361-368.

612. Workman JL, Abmayr SM, Cromlish WA et al. Transcriptional regulation by the immediate early protein of pseudorabies virus during in vitro nucleosome assembly. Cell 1987; 51:613-62.

616. Gross DS, Garrard WT. Nuclease hypersensitive sites in chromatin. Ann Rev Biochem 1988; 57:159-97.

617. Ip YT, Jackson V, Meier J et al. The separation of transcriptionally engaged genes. J Biol Chem 1988; 263:14044-14502.

618. Lorch Y, LaPointe JW, Kornberg RD. On the displacement of histones from DNA by transcription. Cell 1988; 55:743-744.

619. Croston G, Kerrigan L, Lira L et al. Sequence specific anti-repression of histone H1-mediated inhibition of basal RNA polymerase II transcription. Science 1991; 251:643-649.

620. Nacheva G, Guschin DY, Preobrazhenskaya OV et al. Change in the pattern of histone binding to DNA upon transcriptional activation. Cell 1989; 58:27-36.

621. Felsenfeld G. Chromatin as an essential part of the transcriptional mechanism. Nature 1992; 355:219-224.

622. Knezetic JA, Luse DS. The presence of nucleosomes on a DNA template prevents initiation by RNA polymerase II in vitro. Cell 1986; 45:95-104.

623. Lorch Y, LaPointe JW, Kornberg RD. Nucleosomes inhibit the initiation of transcription but allow chain elongation with the displacement of histones. Cell 1987; 49:203-210.

624. Matsui T. Transcription of the adenovirus 2 major late and peptide IX genes under conditions of in vitro nucleosome assembly. Molec Cell Biol 1987; 7:1401-1408.

625. Workman JL, Roeder RG. Binding of transcription factor TFIID to the major late promoter during in vitro nucleosome assembly potentiates subsequent initiation by RNA polymerase II. Cell 1987; 51:613-622.

626. Workman JL, Roeder RG, Kingston RE. An upstream transcription factor, USF (MLTF) facilitates the formation of pre-initiation complexes during in vitro chromatin assembly. EMBO J 1990; 9:1299-1308.

627. Kamakaka RT, Bulger M, Kadonaga JT. Potentiation of RNA polymerase

II transcription by Gal4-VP16 during but not after DNA replication and chromatin assembly. Gen Develop 1993; 7:1779-1795.

628. Meisterernst M, Horikoshi M, Roeder RG. Recombinant yeast TFIID a general transcription factor, mediates activation by the gene-specific factor USF in a chromatin assembly assay. Proc Natl Acad Sci 1990; 87:9153-9157.

629. Shimamura A, Sapp M, Rodriguez-Campos A et al. Histone H1 represses transcription from mini chromosomes assembled in vitro. Molec Cell Biol 1989; 9:5573-5584.

630. Yuan R, Bohan C, Shiao FCH et al. Activation of HIV LTR-directed expression: Analysis with pseudorabies virus immediate early gene. Virology 1989; 172:92-99.

631. Levy A, Noll M. Chromatin fine structure of active and repressed genes. Nature 1981; 289:198-203.

632. Wu C, Wong Y-C, Elgin SCR. The chromatin structure of specific genes II. Disruption of chromatin structure during gene activity. Cell 1979; 16:807-814.

633. Pederson DS, Thomas F, Simpson RT. Core particle, fiber, and transcriptionally active chromatin structure. Ann Rev Cell Biol 1986; 2:117-147.

634. Levinger L, Varshavsky A. Selective arrangement of ubiquitinated and D1 protein-containing nucleosomes within the Drosophila genome. Cell 1982; 28: 375-385.

635. Corthesy B, Leonard P, Wahli W. Transcriptional potentiation of the vitellogenin B1 promoter by a combination of both nucleosome assembly and transcription factors: an in vitro dissection. Molec Cell Biol 1990; 10:3926-3933.

636. Schild C, Claret F-X, Wahli W et al. A nucleosome-dependent static loop potentiates estrogen-regulated transcription from the Xenopus vitellogenin B1 promoter in vitro. EMBO J 1993; 12:423-433.

637. van Holde K. The omnipotent nucleosome. Nature 1992; 362:111-112.

638. Elgin SCR. The formation and function of DNase I hypersensitive sites in the process of gene activation. J Biol Chem 1988; 263:19259-19262.

639. Perlmann T. Glucocorticoid receptor DNA-binding specificity is increased by the organization of DNA in nucleosomes. Proc Natl Acad Sci 1992; 89:3884-3888.

640. Li Q, Wrange O. Translational positioning of a nucleosomal glucocorticoid response element modulates glucocorticoid receptor affinity. Gen Develop 1993; 7:2471-2482.

641. Buetti E, Kuhnel B. Distinct sequence elements involved in the glucocorticoid regulation of the mouse mammary tumor virus promoter identified by linker scanning mutagenesis. J Molec Biol 1986; 190:379-389.

642. Cordingly MG, Riegel AT, Hager GL. Steroid-dependent interaction of transcription factors with the inducible promoter of mouse mammary tumor virus in vivo. Cell 1987; 48:261-270.

643. Rosenfeld PJ, Kelly TJ. Purification of nuclear factor I by DNA recognition site affinity chromatography. J Biol Chem 1986; 261:1398-1408.

644. Cordingly MG, Hager GL. Binding of multiple factors to the MMTV promoter in erode and fractionated nuclear extracts. Nucleic Acid Res 1988; 16:609-628.

645. Richard-Foy H, Hager GL. Sequence specific positioning of nucleosomes over the steroid-inducible MMTV promoter. EMBO J 1987; 6:2321-2328.

646. Perlmann T, Wrange O. Specific glucocortoid receptor binding to DNA reconstituted in a nucleosome. EMBO J 1988; 7:3073-3079.

647. Pina B, Bruggemeir U, Beato M. Nucleosome positioning modulated accessibility of regulatory proteins to the mouse mammary tumor virus promoter. Cell 1990; 60:719-731.

648. Archer TK, Lefebvre P, Wolford RG et al. Transcription factor loading on the MMTV promoter: A bimodal mechanism for promoter activation. Science 1992; 255:1573-1576.

649. Lee H-L, Archer TK. Nucleosome-mediated disruption of transcription factor-chromatin initiation complexes at the mouse mammary tumor virus long terminal repeat in vivo. Molec Cell Biol 1994; 14:32-41.

650. Almouzni G, Wolffe AP. Replication-coupled chromatin assembly is required for the repression of basal transcription in vivo. Gen Develop 1993; 7:2033-2047.

651. Yoshinaga SK, Peterson CL, Herskowitz I et al. Roles of SWI1, SWI2, and SWI3 proteins for transcriptional enhancement by steroid receptors. Science 1992; 258:1598-1604.

652. Bruggemeier U, Rogge L, Winnacker E-L et al. Nuclear factor I acts as a transcription factor on the MMTV promoter but competes with steroid hormone receptors for DNA binding. EMBO J 1990; 7:2233-2239.

653. Verdin E, Paras Jr P, Van Lint C. Chromatin disruption in the promoter of human immunodeficiency virus type 1 during transcriptional activation. EMBO J 1993; 12:3249-3259.

654. Clouse KA, Powell D, Washington I et al. Monokine regulation of HIV-1 expression in a chronically infected human T cell clone. J Immunol 1989; 142:431-438.

655. Han M, Grunstein M. Nucleosome loss activates yeast downstream promoters in vivo. Cell 1988; 55:1137-1145.

656. Han M, Kim U-J, Kayne P et al. Depletion of histone H4 and nucleosomes activates the PHO5 gene in Saccharomyces cerevisiae. EMBO J 1988; 7:2221-2228.

657. Bergman LW. A DNA fragment containing the upstream activator sequence determines nucleosome positioning of the transcriptionally repressed PHO5 gene of *Saccharomyces cerevisiae*. Molec Cell Biol 1986; 6:2298-2304.

658. Schmid A, Fascher C-F, Horz W. Nucleosome disruption at the yeast PHO5 promoter upon PHO5 induction occurs in the absence of DNA replication. Cell 1992; 71:853-864.

659. Reik A, Schytz G, Stewart AF. Glucocorticoids are required for establishment and maintenance of a alteration in chromatin structure: induction leads to a reversible disruption of nucleosomes over an enhancer. EMBO J 1991; 10:2569-2576.

660. Johnston M. A model fungal gene regulation mechanisms: the GAL genes of saccharomyes cervisiae. Microbiol Rev 1987; 51:458-476.

661. Lohr D, Torchia T, Hopper J. The regulatory protein GAL80 is a determinant of the chromatin structure of the yeast GAL1-10 control region. J Biol Chem 1987; 262:15589-15597.

662. Lohr D. Chromatin structure and regulation of the eukaryotic regulatory

gene GAL80. Proc Natl Acad Sci USA 1993; 90:10628-10632.

663. Workman JL, Kingston RE. Nucleosome core displacement in vitro via a metastable transcription factor-nucleosome complex. Science 1992; 258:1780-1783.

664. Morse RH. Nucleosome disruption by transcription factor binding in yeast. Science 1993; 262:1563-1565.

665. Axelrod JD, Reagan MS, Majors J. GAL4 disrupts a repressing nucleosome during activation of GAL1 transcription in vivo. Gen Develop 1993; 7:857-869.

666. Ito M, Sharma A, Lee A et al. Cell cycle regulation of H2b histone octamer DNA binding activity in Chinese hamster lung fibroblasts. Molec Cell Biol 1989; 9:869-873.

667. Krude T, Knippers R. Transfer of nucleosomes from parental to replicated chromatin. Molec Cell Biol 1991; 11:6257-6267.

668. Simpson R. Nucleosome positioning can affect the function of a cis-acting DNA element in vivo. Nature 1990; 343:387-389.

669. Croston GE, Kadonaga JT. Role of chromatin structure in the regulation of transcription by RNA polymerase II. Curr Opin Cell Biol 1993; 5:417-423.

670. Turner BM. Decoding the nucleosome. Cell 1993; 75:5-8.

671. Pfeffer U, Ferrari N, Tosetti F et al. Histone hyperacetylation is induced in chick erythrocyte nuclei during reactivation in heterokaryons. Exp Cell Res 1988; 178:25-30.

672. Vidali G, Boffa L, Mann RS et al. Reversible effects of Na-Butyrate on histone acetylation. Biochem Biophys Res Comm 1978; 82:223-227.

673. Profumo A, Querzola F, Vidali G. Core histones acetylation during lymphocyte activation. FEBS Letter 1989; 250:297-300.

674. Johnson L, Kayne P, Kahn E et al. Genetic evidence for an interaction between SIR3 and histone H4 in the repression of the silent mating loci in Saccharomyces cerevisiae. Proc Natl Acad Sci USA 1990; 87:6286-6290.

675. Park E-C, Szostak J. Point mutations in the yeast histone H4 gene prevent silencing of the silent mating locus HML. Molec Cell Biol 1990; 10:4932-4934.

676. Boffa LC, Vidali G, Mann RS et al. Suppression of histone deacetylation in vivo and in vitro by sodium butyrate. J Biol Chem 1978; 253:3364-3366.

677. Cousens LS, Gallwitz D, Alberts BM. Different accessibilities in chromatin to histone acetylase. J Biol Chem 1979; 254:1716-1723.

678. Krajewski WA, Luchnik AN. Relationship of histone acetylation to DNA topiology and transcription. Molec Gen Genet 1991; 230:442-448.

679. Stadel J, Poksay K, Nakada M et al. Regulation of β-adenoceptor number and subtype in 3T3-L1 preadipocytes by sodium butyrate. Euro J Pharm 1987; 143:35-44.

680. Kruh J. Effects of sodium butyrate a new pharmacological agent, on cells in culture. Molec Cell Biochem 1982; 42: 65-82.

681. Long CW, Suk WA, Snead RM et al. Cell cycle-specific enhancement of type C virus activation by sodium n-butyrate. Cancer Res 1987; 40:203-210.

682. Darzynkiewicz Z, Carter SP. Thermal stability of nucleosomes studied in situ by flow cytometry: Effect of ionic strength and n-butyrate. Exp Cell

Res 1989; 180:551-556.

683. Norton V B Imai P, Yau et al. Histone acetylation reduces nucleosome core particle linking number change. Cell 1989; 57: 449-457.

684. Oliva R D P Bazett-Jones L Locklear et al. Histone hyperacetylation can induce unfolding of the nucleosome core particle. Nucl Acid Res 1990; 18: 2739-2747.

685. Laughlin MA, Zeichner S, Kolson D et al. Sodium butyrate treatment of cells latently infected with HIV-1 results in the expression of unspliced viral RNA. Virology 1993; 196:496-505.

686. Bohan C, Yerk D, Srinivasan A. Sodium butyrate activates human immunodeficiency virus long terminal repeat-directed expression. Biochem Biophys Res Comm 1987; 148:899-905.

687. Bohan C, Robinson RA, Luciw PA et al. Mutational analysis of sodium butyrate inducible elements in the human immunodeficiency virus type I long terminal repeat. Virology 1989; 172:573-583.

688. Contreras-Salazar B, Ehlin-Henriksson B, Klein G et al. Up-regulation of the Epstein Barr Virus (EBV)-encoded membrane protein LMP in the Burkitt's Lymphoma line Daudi after exposure to n-butyrate and after EBV superinfection. J Virol 1990; 64:5441-5447.

689. Shahabuddin M, Volsky B, Kim H et al. Regulated expression of human immunodeficiency virus type 1 in human glial cells: induction of dormant virus. Pathobiol 1992; 60:195-205.

690. Radsak K, Fuhrmann R, Franke RP et al. Induction by sodium butyrate of cytomegalovirus replication in human endothelial cells. Arch Virol 1989; 107:151-158.

691. Cosgrove D, Cox S. Enhancement by theophylline of the butyrate mediated induction of choriogonadotropin alpha subunit in HeLa cells II, Effect of both agents on mRNA turnover. Arch Biochem Biophys 1990; 280:95-102.

692. Luka J, Kallin B, Klein G. Induction of the Epstein-Barr Virus (EBV) cycle in latently infected cells by n-butyrate. Virology 1979; 94:228-231.

693. Ryan M, Higgins P. Cytoarchitecture of Kirsten Sarcoma Virus-transformed rat kidney fibroblasts: butyrate-induced reorganization within the actin microfilament network. J Cell Physiol 1988; 137:25-34.

694. Takano M, Rhoads DB, Isselbacher KJ. Sodium butyrate increases glucose transporter expression in LLC-PK1 cells. Proc Natl Acad Sci USA 1988; 85:8072-8075.

695. Tang D-C, Taylor M. Transcriptional activation of the adenine phosphoribosyltransferase promoter by an upstream butyrate-induced moloney murine sarcoma virus enhancer-promoter element. J Virol 1990; 64:2907-2911.

696. McKnight GS, Hager L, Palmiter RD. Butyrate and related inhibitors of histone deacetylation block the induction of egg white genes by steroid hormones. Cell 1980; 22:469-477.

697. Plesko MM, Hargrove JL, Granner DK et al. Inhibition by sodium butyrate of enzyme induction by glucocorticoids and dibutyryl cyclic AMP. J Biol Chem 1983; 258(22): 13738-13744.

698. Bresnick EH, John S, Bernard DS et al. Glucocorticoid receptor-dependent disruption of a specific nucleosome on the mouse mammary tumor virus promoter is prevented by sodium butyrate. Proc Natl Acad Sci USA

1990; 87:3977-3981.

699. Golub EI, Li G, Volsky DJ. Induction of dormant HIV-1 by sodium butyrate: Involvement of the TATA box in the activation of the HIV-1 LTR. AIDS 1991; 5:663-668.

700. Laughlin, MA, Chang, GY, Oakes, JW, Gonzalez-Scarano F, Pomerantz RJ. Sodium butyrate stimulation of HIV-1 gene expression: a novel mechanism of induction independent of NF-κB submitted 1994.

701. Bradbury EM. Reversible histone modifications and the chromosome cell cycle. BioEssays 1992; 14:9-16.

702. Bode J, Maass K. Chromatin domain surrounding the human interferon β gene as defined by scaffold attached regions. Biochem 1988; 27: 4707-4711.

703. Gasser SM, Laemmle UK. Cohabitation of scaffold binding regions with upstream/enhancer elements of three developmentally regulated genes of D, melanogaster. Cell 1986; 46:521-530.

704. Klehr D, Schlake T, Maass K et al. Scaffold attached regions (SAR elements) mediate transcriptional effects due to butyrate. Biochem 1992; 31:3222-3229.

705. McKnight RA, Shamay A, Sankaran L et al. Matrix-attachment regions can impart position-independent regulation of a tissue specific gene in transgenic mice. Proc Natl Acad Sci USA 1992; 89:6943-6947.

706. Phi-Van L, von Kries JP, Ostertag W et al. The chicken lysozyme 5' matrix attachment region increases transcription from a heterologous promoter in heterologous cells and dampens position effects on the expression of transfected genes. Molec Cell Biol 1990; 10: 2302-2307.

707. Schaak J, Ho WY, Freimuth P et al. Adenovirus terminal protein mediated both nuclear matrix association and efficient transcription of adenovirus DNA. Gen Develop 1990; 4:1197-1208.

708. Steif A, Winter DM, Stratling WH et al. A nuclear DNA attachment element mediates elevated and position independent gene activity. Nature 1989; 341:343-345.

709. Brinster RL et al. Somatic expression of herpes thymidine kinase in mice following injection of a fusion gene into eggs. Cell 1981; 27:223-231.

710. Kucherlapati R, Skoultchi AJ. Introduction of purified genes into mammalian cells. Crit Rev Biochem 1984; 16:349-381.

711. Palmiter RD, Brinster RL. Transgenic mice. Cell 1985; 41:343-345.

712. Razin SV, Petrov P, Hancock R. Precise localization of the α-globin gene cluster within one of the 20-to 300-kilobase DNA fragments released by cleavage of chicken chromosomal DNA at topoisomerase II sites in vivo: Evidence that the fragments are DNA loops or domains. Proc Natl Acad Sci USA 1991; 88:8515-8519.

713. Lowrey CH, Bodine DM, Nienhuis AW. Mechanism of DNase I hypersensitive site formation within the human globin control region. Proc Natl Acad Sci USA 1992; 89:1143-1147.

714. Talbot D, Collis P, Antoniou M et al. A dominant control region from the human β-globin locus conferring integration site-independent gene expression. Nature 1989; 338:352-355.

715. Farache G, Razin SV, Rzeszowska-Wolny J et al. Mapping of structural and transcription-related matrix attachment sites in the α-globin gene domain of avian erythroblasts and erythrocytes. Molec Cell Biol 1990;

10:5349-5358.

716. Reitman M, Felsenfeld G. Developmental regulation of topoisomerase II sites and DNase I-hypersensitive sites in the chicken β-globin locus. Molec Cell Biol 1990; 10:2774-2786.

717. Caterina JJ, Ciavatta DJ, Donze D et al. Multiple elements in human β-globin locus control region 5' HS 2 are involved in enhancer activity and position-independent, transgene expression. Nucl Acid Res 1994; 22:1006-1011.

718. Philipsen S, Talbot D, Fraser P et al. The β-globin dominant control region: hypersensitive site 2. EMBO J 1990; 9:2159-2167.

719. Morley BJ, Abbott CA, Sharpe JA et al. A single β-globin locus control region element (5' hypersensitive site 2) is sufficient for developmental regulation of human globin genes in transgenic mice. Molec Cell Biol 1992; 12:2057-2066.

720. Jankelevich S, Kolman JL, Bodnar JW et al. A nuclear matrix attachment region organizes the Epstein-Barr viral plasmid in Raji cells into a single DNA domain. EMBO J 1992; 11:1165-1176.

721. Schaack J, Ho WY, Freimuth P et al. Adenovirus terminal protein mediates both nuclear matrix association and efficient transcription of adenovirus DNA. Gen Dev 1990; 4:1197-1200.

722. Leonard MW, Patient RK. Evidence for torsional stress in transcriptionally activated chromatin. Molec Cell Biol 1991; 11:6128-6138.

723. Liu L. DNA topoisomerase poisons as anti-tumor drugs. Ann Rev Biochem 1989; 58:351-75.

724. Kroeger PE, Rowe TC. Analysis of topoisomerase I and II cleavage sites on the *Drosophila* actin and Hsp70 Heat Shock. Genes Biochem 1992; 31:2492-2501.

725. Porter SE, Champoux JJ. Mapping in vivo topoisomerase I sites on simian virus 40 DNA: Asymmetric distribution of sites on replicating molecules. Molec Cell Biol 1989; 9:541-550.

726. Bojanowski K, Lelievre S, Markovits J et al. Suramin is an inhibitor of DNA topoisomerase II in vitro and in Chinese hamster fibrosarcoma cells Proc Natl Acad Sci USA 1992; 89: 3025-3029.

727. Balzarini J, Mitsuya H, De Clerq E et al. Comparative inhibitory effects of suramin and other selected compounds on the infectivity and replication of human T-cell lymphotrophic virus (HTLV-III)/lymphadenopathy-associated virus (LAV). Int J Cancer 1986; 37:451-457.

728. Mitsuya H, Popovic M, Yarchoan R et al. Suramin protection of T cells in vitro against infectivity and cytopathic effect of HTLV-III. Science 1984; 226:172-174.

729. Broder S, Collins JM, Markham PD et al. Effects of suramin on HTLV-III/LAV infection presenting as Kaposi's sarcoma or AIDS related complex: Clinical pharmacology and repression of virus replication in vivo. Lancet 627-630, 1985.

730. Levine AM, Gill PS, Cohen J et al. Suramin antiviral therapy in the acquired immunodeficiency syndrome. Ann Int Med 1986; 105: 32-37.

731. Cheson BD, Levine AM, Mildvan D et al. Suramin therapy in AIDS and related disorders. JAMA 1987; 258:1347-1351.

732. Kaplan LD, Wolfe PR, Volberding PA et al. Lack of response to suramin in patients with AIDS and AIDS-related complex. Am J Med 1987; 82:

615-620.

733. LeGuenno BM, Barabe P, Griffet PA et al. HIV-1 and HIV-1 AIDS cases in Senegal: Clinical patterns and immunological perturbations. J AIDS 1991; 4:421-427.

734. Lisse IM, Poulsen A-G, Aaby P et al. Immunodeficiency in HIV-1 infections: A community study from Guinea-Bissau. AIDS 1990; 4:1263-1266.

735. Pepin J, Morgan G, Dunn D et al. HIV-1-induced immunosuppression among asymptomatic West African prostitutes: Evidence that HIV-1 is pathogenic, but less so than HIV-1. AIDS 1991; 5:1165-1172.

736. Kestens K, Brattegaard K, Adjorlolo G et al. Immunological comparison of HIV-1 and HIV-1- and dually-reactive women delivery in Abidjan, Cote d'Ivoire. AIDS 1992; 6:803-807.

737. Egboga A, Corrah T, Todd A et al. Immunological findings in African patients with pulmonary tuberculosis and HIV-2 infection. AIDS 1992; 6:1045-1046.

738. Marlink R, Kanki P, Thior I et al. Reduced rate of disease development after HIV-1 infection as compared to HIV-1. Science 1994; 265:1587-1590.

739. Kawamura M, Yamazaki S, Ishikawa K et al. HIV-1 in West Africa in 1966. Lancet 1989; 1:385.

740. Le Guenno B. HIV-1 and HIV-1: Two ancient viruses for a new disease? Trans R Soc Trop Med Hyg 1989; 83:847.

741. Del Mistro A, Chotard J, Hall AJ et al. HIV-1 and HIV-2 seroprevalence rates in mother-child pairs living in the Gambia (West Africa). J AIDS 1992; 5:1924.

742. Pousen A-G, Kvinedal BB, Aaby P et al. Lack of evidence of vertical transmission of human immunodeficiency virus type 2 in a sample of the general population in Bissau. J AIDS 1992; 5:25-30.

743. De Cock KM, Odehouri K, Colebunders RL et al. A comparison of HIV-1 and HIV-2-infections in hospitalized patients in Abidjan, Cote d'Ivoire. AIDS 1990; 4:443-448.

744. Poulsen AG, Kvinesdal B, Aaby P et al. Prevalence of and mortality from human immunodeficiency virus type 2 in Bissau, West Africa. Lancet 1989; 1:827-831.

745. Wilkins A, Ricard D, Todd J et al. The epidemiology of HIV infection in a rural area of Guinea-Bissau. AIDS 1993; 7:1119-1122.

746. DeCock KM, Brun-Vezinet F, Soro B. HIV-1 and HIV-2 infections and AIDS in West Africa. AIDS 1991; 5(suppl):S21-S28.

747. Savarit D, De Cock KM, Schutz R et al. A risk of HIV infection from transfusion with blood negative for HIV antibody in a West African city. BMJ 1992; 305:498-502.

748. Simon F, Matheron S, Tamalet C et al. Cellular and plasma viral load in patients infected with HIV-2. AIDS 1993; 7:1411-1417.

749. Report of a Consensus Workshop, Sienna, Italy, January 17-18, 1992: Factors involved in mother-to-child transmission of HIV. J AIDS 1992; 5:1019-1029.

750. Emerman M, Guyader M, Montagnier L et al. The specificity of the human immunodeficiency virus type 2 transactivator is different from that of human immunodeficiency virus type 1. EMBO J 1987; 6:3755-60.

751. Berkhout B, Gatignol A, Silver J et al. Efficient transactivation by the

HIV-2 *tat* protein requires a duplicated TAR RNA structure. Nucl Acid Res 1990; 18:1839-46.

752. Echetebu CO, Rice AP. Mutational analysis of the amino and carboxy termini of the HIV-2 *tat* protein. J AIDS 1993; 6:550-557.

753. Echetebu CO, Rhim H, Herrman CH et al. Construction and characterization of a potent HIV-1 *tat* transdominant mutant protein. J AIDS 1994; 7:655-664.

754. Arya SK. Human immunodeficiency virus type 2 (HIV-2) transactivator (*tat*): functional domains and the search for transdominant negative mutants. AIDS Res and Human Retrov 1993; 9:839-848.

755. Chang Y-N, Jeang K-T. The basic RNA-binding domain of HIV-2 *Tat* contributes to preferential transactivation of a Tar2-containing LTR. Nucl Acids Res 1992; 20:5465-5472.

756. Elangovan B, Subramanian T, Chinnadurai G. Functional comparison of the basic domains of the *tat* proteins of human immunodeficiency virus types 1 and 2 in transactivation. J Virol 1992; 66:2031-2036.

757. Rhim H, Rice AP. TAR RNA-binding properties and relative transactivation activities of human immunodeficiency virus type 1 and 2 *tat* proteins. J Virol 1993; 67:1110-1121.

758. Fenrick R, Malim MH, Hauber J et al. Functional analysis of the *tat* trans activator of human immunodeficiency virus type 2. J Virol 1989; 63:5006-5012.

759. Tong-Starksen SE, Baur A, Lu X-B et al. Second exon of *tat* of HIV-2 is required for optimal transactivation of HIV-1 and HIV-2 LTRs. Virology 1993; 195:826-830.

760. Rhim H, Rice AP. Functional significance of the dinucleotide bulge in stem-loop 1 and stem-loop 2 of HIV-1 Tar RNA. Virology 1994; 202:202-211.

761. Berkhout B, Gatignol A, Silver J et al. Efficient trans-activation by the HIV-1 *Tat* protein requires a duplicated TAR RNA structure. Nucl Acids Res 1990; 18:1839-1846.

762. Le S-Y, Malim MH, Cullen BR et al. A highly conserved RNA folding region coincident with the *Rev* response element of primate immunodeficiency viruses. Nucl Acids Res 1990; 18:1613-1623.

763. Sakai H, Siomi H, Shida H et al. A functional comparison of transactivation by human retrovirus *rev* and *rex* genes. J Virol 1990; 64:5833-5839.

764. Luciw PA, Shacklett BL. Molecular biology of the human and simian immunodeficiency viruses. In: HIV Molecular Organization, Pathogenicity and Treatment. Elsevier Science Publishers B.V, 1993:123-151.

765. Hirsch VM, Myers G, Johnson PR. Genetic diversity and phylogeny of primate lentiviruses. In: HIV Molecular Organization, Pathogenicity and Treatment. Elsevier Science Publishers B.V, 1993:221-240.

766. Leiden JM, Wang C-Y, Petryniak B et al. A novel Ets-related transcription factor, Elf-1, binds to human immunodeficiency virus type 2 regulatory elements that are required for inducible trans-activation in T cells. J Virol 1992; 66:5890-5897.

767. Markovitz DM, Hannibal M, Perez VL et al. Differential regulation of human immunodeficiency viruses (HIVs): A specific regulatory element in HIV-2 responds to stimulation of the T-cell antigen receptor. Proc

Natl Acad Sci USA 1990; 87:9098-9102.

768. Markovitz DM, Smith M, Hilfinger JM et al. Activation of the human immunodeficiency virus type 2 enhancer is dependent on purine box and κB regulatory elements. J Virol 1992; 66:5479-5484.

769. Hilfinger J, Clark N, Smith M et al. Differential regulation of the human immunodeficiency virus type 2 enhancer in monocytes at various stages of differentiation. J Virol 1993; 67:4448-4453.

770. Hannibal MC, Markovitz DM, Clark N et al. Differential activation of human immunodeficiency virus type 1 and 2 transcription by specific T-cell activation signals. J Virol 1993; 67:5035-5040.

771. Hirsch VM, Johnson PR. Pathogenic diversity of simian immunodeficiency viruses. Virus Res 1994; 32:183-203.

772. Allan JS. Pathogenic properties of simian immunodeficiency viruses in non-human primates. In: Koff W et al, eds. Annual Review of AIDS Research. Vol 1 M. Dekker, NY, 1991:191-206.

773. Gravell M, London WT, Hamilton RS et al. Infection of macaque monkeys with simian immunodeficiency virus from African green monkeys: virulence and activation of latent infection. J Med Primatol 1989; 18:247-256.

774. Johnson RP, Goldstein S, London WT et al. Molecular clones of SIVsm and SIV agm: Experimental infection of macaques and African green monkeys. J Med Primatol 1990; 19:279-286.

775. Honjo S, Narita T, Kobayashi R et al. Experimental infection of African green monkeys and cynomologous monkeys with a SIVagm strain isolated from a healthy African green monkey. J Med Primatol 1990; 19:9-20.

776. Hartung S, Boller K, Cichutek K et al. Quantitation of a lentivirus in its natural host: simian immunodeficiency virus in African green monkeys. J Virol 1992; 66:2143-2149.

777. Sakuragi J-I, Fukasawa M, Shibata R et al. Functional analysis of long terminal repeats derived from four strains of simian immunodeficiency virus SIVagm in relation to other primate lentiviruses. Virology 1991; 185:455-459.

778. Saksela K, Muchmore E, Girard M et al. High viral load in lymph nodes and latent human immunodeficiency virus (HIV) in peripheral blood cells of HIV-1-infected chimpanzees. J Virol 1993; 67:7423-7427.

779. Letvin NL, Eaton KA, Adrich WR et al. Acquired immunodeficiency syndrome in a colony of macaque monkeys. Proc Natl Acad Sci USA 1983; 80:2718-2722.

780. Hunt RD, Blake BJ, Chalifoux LV et al. Transmission of naturally occurring lymphoma in macaque monkeys. Proc Natl Acad Sci USA 1983; 80:5085-5089.

781. Letvin NL, Aldrich WR, King NW et al. Experimental transmission of macaque AIDS by means of inoculation of macaque lymphoma tissue. Lancet 1983; 2:599-602.

782. Letvin NL, Daniel MD, Sehgal PK et al. Induction of AIDS-like disease in macaque monkeys with T-cell tropic retrovirus STLV-III. Science 1985; 230:71-73.

783. Daniel MD, Letvin NL, King NW. Isolation of T-cell tropic HTLV-III-like retrovirus from macaques. Science 1985; 228:1201-1204.

784. Reimann KA, Tenner-Racz K, Racz P et al. Immunopathogenic events in acute infection of rhesus monkeys with simian immunodeficiency virus of macaques. J Virol 1994; 68:2362-2370.

785. Schwartz D, Sharma U, Busch M et al. Absence of recoverable infectious virus and unique immune responses in an asymptomatic HIV + long term survivor. AIDS & Human Retrovir 1994 (In Press).

786. Fultz PN, McClure HM, Anderson DC et al. Identification and biologic characterization of an acutely lethal variant of simian immunodeficiency virus from sooty mangabeys (SIV/SMM). AIDS Res Hum Retrov 1989; 5:397-409.

787. Lewis MG, Zack PM, Elkins WR. Infection of rhesus and cynomolgous macaques with a rapidly fatal SIV (SIV$_{SMM/PBj}$) isolate from sooty mangabeys. AIDS Res and Human Retroviruses 1992; 8:1631-1639.

788. Israel ZR, Dean GA, Maul DH et al. Early pathogenesis of disease caused by (SIV$_{SMM/PBj-14}$) molecular clone 1.9 in macaques. AIDS Res and Human Retrov 1993; 9:277-286.

789. Birx DL, Lewis MG, Vahey M et al. Association of interleukin-6 in the pathogenesis of acutely fatal SIV$_{SMM/PBj-14}$ in pigtailed macaques. AIDS Res and Human Retrov 1993; 9:1123-1129.

790. Courgnaud V, Laure F, Fultz PN et al. Genetic differences accounting for evolution and pathogenicity of simian immunodeficiency virus from a sooty mangabey monkey after cross-species transmission to a pigtailed macaque. J Virol 1992; 66:414-419.

791. Novembre FJ, Johnson RP, Lewis MjG et al. Multiple viral determinants contribute to pathogenicity of the acutely lethal simian immunodeficiency virus SIV$_{SMM/PBj}$ variant. J Virol 1993; 67:2466-2474.

792. Marthas ML, Ramos RA, Lohman BL et al. Viral determinants of simian immunodeficiency virus (SIV) virulence n rhesus macaques assessed by using attentuated and pathogenic molecular clones of SIVmac. J Virol 1993; 67:6047-6055.

793. Kestler H, Kodama T, Ringler D et al. Induction of AIDS in rhesus monkeys by molecularly cloned simian immunodeficiency virus. Science 1990; 248:1109-112.

794. Marthas ML, Banapour B, Sutjipto S et al. Rhesus macaques inoculated with molecularly clones simian immunodeficiency virus. J Med Primatol 1989; 18:311-319.

795. Winandy S, Boris R, Li Y et al. Nuclear factors that bind two regions important to transcriptional activity of the Simian immunodeficiency virus long terminal repeat. J Virol 1992; 66:5216-5223.

796. Bellas RE, Hopkins N, Li Y. The NF-κB binding site is necessary for efficient replication of Simian immunodeficiency virus of macaques in primary macrophages but not in T cells in vitro. J Virol 1993; 67:2908-2913.

797. Miyoshi I, Ohtuki Y, Fujishita M et al. Detection of type-C virus particles in Japanese monkeys seropositive to adult T-cell leukemia-associated antigens. Gann 1982; 73:848-849.

798. Guo H-G, Wong-Staal F, Gallo RC. Novel viral sequences related to human T-cell leukemia virus in T cells of a seropositive baboon. Science 1984; 223:1195-1197.

799. Yamaoto N, Hinuma Y, Sur Hausen H et al. African green monkeys are

infected with adult T-cell leukemia virus or a closely related agent. Lancet 1983; i:240.

800. Sugamura K and Hinuma Y Human retroviruses: HTLV-I and HTLV-II. In: Levy JA, ed. The Retroviridae, vol 2 1993. Plenum Press, New York.

801. Hayami M Simian T-cell leukemia virus (STLV-I):HTLV-I related virus in non-human primates. In: Takatsuki T et al, eds. The Advances in ATL and HTLV-I Research, 1991; Plenum Press New York.

803. Koralnik IJ, Boeri E, Saxinger WC et al. Phylogenetic associations of human and simian T-cell leukemia/lymphoma virus type I strains: Evidence for interspecies transmission. J Virol 1994; 68:2693-2707.

804. Paine E, Garcia J, Philpott TC et al. Limited sequence variation in human T-lymphotropic virus type 1 isolates from North American and African patients. Virology 1991; 182:111-123.

805. Homma T, Kanki PJ, Hunt RD et al. Lymphoma in macaques: association with virus of human T lymphotropic family. Science 1984; 225:716-718.

806. Tsujimoto H Noda, Y, Ishikawa K et al. Development of adult T-cell leukemia-like diseases in an African green monkey associated with clonal integration of simian T-cell leukemia virus type 1. Cancer Res 1986; 47:269-274.

807. Nakano S, Ando Y, Ichijo M et al. Search for possible routes of vertical and horizontal transmission of adult T-cell leukemia virus. Gann 1984; 75:1044

808. Ando Y, Nakano S, Saito K et al. Transmission of adult T-cell leukemia retrovirus (HTLV-I) from mother to child: Comparison of bottle-with breast-fed babies. Jpn J Cancer Res 1987; 78:322.

809. Ando Y, Saito K, Nakano S et al. Bottle-feeding can prevent transmission of HTLV-I from mothers to their babies. J Infect 1989; 19:25.

810. Hino S, Yamaguchi K, Katamine S et al. Mother-t-child transmission of human T-cell leukemia virus type I. Jpn J Cancer Res 1985; 76:474-480.

811. Okochi K, Sato JH, Hinuma Y. A retrospective study on transmission of adult T-cell leukemia virus by blood transfusion: seroconversion in recipients. Vox Sang 1984; 46:245.

812. Zella D, Mori L, Sala M et al. HTLV-II infection in Italian drug abusers. Lancet 1990; 336:575.

813. Lee H, Swanson P, Shorty VS et al. High rate of HTLV-II infection in seropositive IV drug abusers in New Orleans. Science 1989; 244:471-475.

814. Seiki M, Hattori S, Hirayama Y et al. Human adult T-cell leukemia virus: complete nucleotide sequence of the provirus genome integrated in leukemia cell. Proc Natl Acad Sci USA 1983; 80:3618-3622.

815. Shimotohno K, Takehashi Y, Shimizu N et al. Complete nucleotide sequence of an infectious clone of human T-cell leukemia virus type II: an open reading frame for the protease gene. Proc Natl Acad Sci USA 1985; 82:31013105.

816. Felber BK, Paskalis H, Kleinman-Ewing C et al. The pX protein of HTLV-I is a transcriptional activator of its long terminal repeat. Science 1985; 229:675-678.

817. Sodroski JG, Rosen CA, Haseltine WA. Trans-acting transcriptional activation of the long terminal repeat of human T lymphotropic viruses in

infected cells. Science 1984; 225:381-421.

818. Nyborg JK, Dynan WS, Chen, ISY et al. Binding of host-cell factors to DNA sequences in the long terminal repeat of human T-cell leukemia virus type I: implications for viral gene expression. Proc Natl Acad Sci USA 1988; 85:1457-1461.

819. Yoshimura T, Fujisawa J-I, Yoshida M. Multiple cDNA slones encoding nuclear proteins that bind to the *tax*-dependent enhancer of HTLV-I: all contain a leucine zipper structure and basic amino acid domain. EMBO J 1990; 9:2537-2542.

820. Fujisawa J-I, Seiki M, Sato M et al. A transcriptional enhancer sequence of HTLV-I is responsible for trans-activation mediated by p40 *tax* of HTLV-I. EMBO J 1986; 5:713-718.

821. Jeang K-T, Boros I, Brady J et al. Characterization of cellular factors that interact with the human T-cell leukemia virus type 1 p40-responsive 21-base pair sequence. J Virol 1988; 62:4499-4509.

822. Shimotohno K, Takano M, Teruuchi T et al. Requirement of multiple copies of a 21 nucleotide sequence in the U3 regions of human T-cell leukemia virus type I and type II long terminal repeats for trans-acting activation of transcription. Proc Natl Acad Sci USA 1986; 83:8112-8226.

823. Ballard DW, Bohnlein E, Lowenthal JW et al. HTLV-I *tax* induces cellular proteins that activate the κB element in the IL-2 receptor α gene. Science 1988; 241:1652-1655.

824. Leung K, Nabel GJ. HTLV-I transactivator induces interleukin 2 receptor expression through an NF-κB like factor. Nature 1988; 333:776-778.

825. Ruben S, Poteat H, Tan T-H et al. Cellular transcription factors and regulation of IL-2 receptor gene expression by HTLV-I *tax* gene product. Science 1988; 241:89-92.

826. Siekevitz M, Josephs SF, Dukovich M et al. Activation of the HIV-1 LTR by T cell mitogens and the trans-activator protein of HTLV-I. Science 1987; 238:1575-1578.

827. Smith MR, Greene WC. Identification of HTLV-I *tax* trans-activator mutants exhibiting novel transcriptional phenotypes. Genes Dev 1990; 4:1875-1885.

828. Rimsky L, Hauber J, Dukovich M et al. Functional replacement of the HIV-1 *rev* protein by the HTLV-I *rex* protein. Nature 1988; 335:738-740.

829. Hanly SM, Rimsky, LT, Malim MH et al. Comparative analysis of the HTLV-I *rex* and HIV-1 *rev* trans-regulatory proteins and their RNA response elements. Genes Dev 1989; 3:1534-1544.

830. Hidaka M, Inoue J, Yoshida M et al. Post-transcriptional regulator (*rex*) of HTLV-I initiates expression of viral structural proteins but suppresses expression of regulatory proteins. EMBO J 1988; 7:519-523.

831. Inoue J-I, Yoshida M, Seike M. Transcriptional (p40x) and post-transcriptional (p27x-III) regulators are required for the expression and replication of human T-cell leukemia virus type I genes. Proc Natl Acad Sci USA 1987; 84:3653-3657.

832. Toyoshima H, Itoh M, Inoue J-I et al. Secondary structure of the human T-cell leukemia virus type I *rex*-responsive element is essential for *rex* regulation of RNA processing and transport of unspliced RNAs. J Virol 1990; 64:2825-2832.

833. Ahmed YF, Hanly SM, Malim MH et al. Structure-function analyses of the HTLV-I *rex* and HIV-1 *rev* RNA responsive elements; insights into the mechanism of *rex* and *rev* action. Genes Dev 1990; 4:1014-1022.

834. Bogerd HP, Huckaby GL, Ahmed YF et al. The type 1 human T-cell leukemia virus (HTLV-I) *rex* trans-activator binds directly to the HTLV-I *rex* and the type 1 human immunodeficiency virus *rev* RNA response element. Proc Natl Acad Sci USA 1991; 88:5704-5708.

835. Unge T, Solomin L, Mellini M et al. The *rex* regulatory protein of human T-cell lymphotropic virus type I binds specifically to its target site within the viral RNA. Proc Natl Acad Sci USA 1991; 88:7145-7149.

836. Zoubak S, Richardson JH, Rynditch A et al. Regional specificity of HTLV-I proviral integration in the human genome. Gene 1994; 143:155-163.

837. zur Hausen H. Viruses in human cancers. Science 1991; 254:1167-1173.

838. Ishida T, Yamamoto K, Omoto K et al. Prevalence of a human retrovirus in native Japanese: Evidence for a possible ancient origin. J Infect 1985; 11:153.

839. Lochelt M, Zentgraf H, Flugel RM. Construction of an infectious DNA clone of the full length human spumaretrovirus genome and mutagenesis of the bel-1 gene. Virology 1991; 184:43-54.

840. Rethwilm A, Baunach G, Netzer K-O et al. Infectious DNA of the human spumaretrovirus. Nucl Acid Res 1990; 4:733-738.

841. Muranyi M, Flugel RM. Analysis of splicing patterns of human spumaretrovirus by polymerase chain reaction reveals complex RNA structures. J Virol 1991; 65:727-735.

842. Keller A, Partin KM, Lochelt M et al. Characterization of the transcriptional trans-activator of human foamy retrovirus. J Virol 1991; 65:2589-2594.

843. Rethwilm A, Erlwein O, Baunach B et al. The transcriptional transactivator of human foamy virus maps to the bel-1 genomic region. Proc Natl Acad Sci USA 1991; 88:941-945.

844. Venkatesh LK, Theodorakis PA, Chinnadurai G. Distinct cis acting regions in U3 regulate trans-activation of the human spumaretrovirus long terminal repeat by the viral bel-1 gene product. Nucl Acid Res 1991; 19:3661-3666.

845. Keller A, Garrett ED, Cullen BR. The bel-1 protein of human foamy virus activates human immunodeficiency virus type 1 gene expression via a novel DNA target site. J Virol 1992; 66:3946-3949.

846. Lee AH, Lee KJ, Cullen BR et al. Transactivation of human immunodeficiency virus type 1 long terminal repeat-directed gene expression by human foamy virus bel-1 protein requires a novel DNA sequence. J Virol 1992; 66:3236-3240.

INDEX

Disease penetrance, 8-9, 85, 92
Disruption, 34, 37, 51, 69, 74-78
Deoxyribonucleic acid (DNA)
 binding affinity, 47, 71
 binding transcriptional factors, 23, 26
  68, 71, 97
 PCR, 13, 16, 92
 topology, 55
DNase, 52, 57, 72, 80
Doerre, 47
Drosophila melanogaster, 22, 69, 80
Duan, 38, 44
Dyspnea, 5

E

E1A, 21, 24-25, 59
Echetebu, 88
Effector domains, 35
Equine infectious anemia virus (EIAV),
 4-5
Electrophoretic mobility shift assay
 (EMSA), 41
ELF, 50
Elgin, 70
Elongation efficiencies, 22-23, 27, 38, 60,
 69, 83
Elongation processes, 22-23
Embretson, 13, 16
Enhancement, 2, 22-25, 39, 41, 43, 45,
 49, 51-54, 57, 60, 65-66, 70, 72,
 74, 79-80, 91, 95
Ensoli, 60
Env, 7, 17-18, 31, 33, 95-97
Environment, 17, 47, 50, 66, 69, 78
Enzymes, 7, 17-18, 46, 61, 77, 80-82, 87
Epidemiology, 5, 86, 97
ERG, 50
ETS, 50-51, 91
Exon tat, 27-28, 87

F

Fankhauser, 36
Fedor, 76
Feline immunodeficiency virus (FIV), 5
Frankel, 28
Function, 14-15, 17-19, 23, 25-38, 40,
 42, 45, 47-48, 52-54, 58, 69, 76,
 88-90, 93, 97-99
Functional domain, 79-80, 90

G

Galactose responsive gene (GAL)
 galactose responsive gene (GAL), 23,
  26, 30, 53, 71-72, 74-76
 GAL3, 75
 GAL4, 23, 26, 30, 53, 75-76
 GAL80, 75-76
 gene regulation, 75-76

Gajdusek, 5
Gaynor, 56, 58
Ghazal, 57
Ghosh, 24
Gislason, 5
Globins, 33, 79
Glucocorticoid receptor, 71
Glucocorticoid responsive element (GRE),
 71, 73
Golub, 78
Gottlieb, 6
Gp41, 12, 17
Gp120, 12, 17, 60
Gp160, 17
Gravell, 92
Green, 1, 3, 8, 23, 28, 92-93, 98
GRF2, 76

H

H1, 66-67, 69
H2A, 66
H2B, 66
H3, 66
H4, 66, 75, 77
H5, 66
H2TF1, 50
Hammarskjold, 33
Hannibal, 91
Hartung, 92
Heat shock, 22-23, 69, 74, 81
Heat shock protein (HSP) 70, 22-23, 69,
 74
HeLa, 21, 29-30, 36-37, 41
Herpes simplex virus (HSV), 1, 57, 59
Heterodimers, 28, 46-47, 49, 52-53
Hexanucleotide loop, 19-20
High mobility group (HMG), 54
Hirsch, 92
Histones, 66-69, 71, 75-78
HIVEN 86A, 50
Homodimers, 26, 46-49
Homosexuals, 6
Hormonal, 4, 40, 54, 70-73, 75, 77-79
Hormonal induction, 4, 72, 75
Host determinants, 65, 67, 69, 71, 73,
 75, 77, 79, 81, 83
Human cytomegalovirus (HCMV), 57-59
Human Immunodeficiency Virus (HIV)
 HIV, 1-3, 5-31, 33-34, 36-48, 50-63,
  65-66, 68-70, 72, 74, 76, 78,
  80-81, 83, 85-99
 HIV-1 long terminal repeat (LTR),
  7, 39, 52, 55, 69, 74
 HIV-1 methylated DNA binding
  protein (HMBP), 41
 HIV gene expression, co-pathogens, 57
 HIV gene structure, 12, 18, 33, 91
 HIV-2, 86
 initiation elements, 24, 39, 42, 45,
  51, 54